Gut Health Cookbook for Women

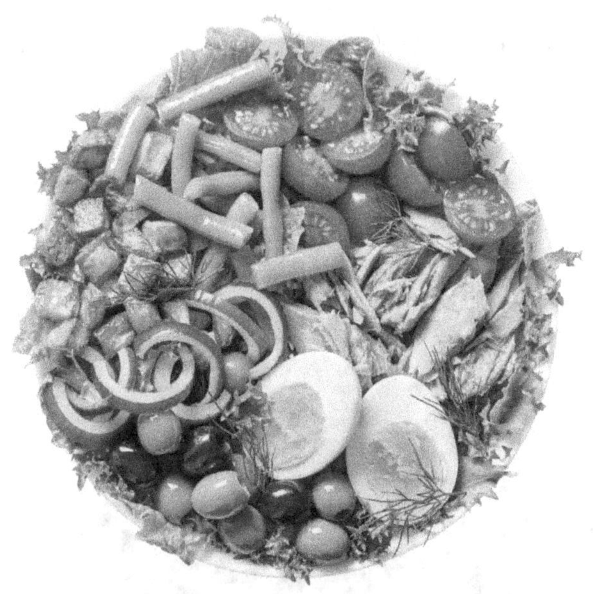

Quick And Easy Delicious and Nutritious Recipes to Reclaim Control Over Your Digestion, Mood, And Boost Overall Health and Meal Plan

Joan G. Milone

Copyright © 2023 by Joan G. Milone

All rights reserved.

This book is written as a source of information only. The information contained in this book is provided in good faith and is believed to be accurate and reliable as of the date of publication. The author does not assume any responsibility for any errors or omissions that may appear.

Scan For More Amazing Cookbooks From Joan

Table of Content

Introduction

Welcome, my reader, to a voyage of tastes and well-being beyond a cookbook's bounds. I am overwhelmed with tremendous enthusiasm and purpose as I write these lines, knowing I am about to begin with you on a revolutionary voyage toward enhanced gut health.

This isn't just another cookbook; it's a sincere investigation of the fundamental link between the food we eat and the complicated world within us—the world of our gut flora. My name is Joan, and I am a professional nutritionist and ardent supporter of holistic health. My purpose as I stand before you through these pages is to lead you down a path where tasty meets nutritious, where the pleasure of eating blends smoothly with the wisdom of sustaining your body from the inside.

This book, sprang from my journey. Like many others, I negotiated life's twists and turns, often ignoring the silent strength within me—the gut. It was a wake-up call, a revelation that the decisions we make in the kitchen have far-reaching consequences beyond flavour and enjoyment. They send shockwaves through our bodies, affecting our vigour, immunity, and general happiness.

Picture this: a watershed points in my life when a seemingly never-ending cycle of exhaustion and intestinal pain compelled me to reconsider my relationship with food. The kitchen, which was once a place of experimentation and fun, became a laboratory for creating meals that satisfied my taste buds and nurtured my stomach.

I discovered the fundamental relationship between intestinal health and general well-being when immersed in the fragrant dance of spices and the sizzle of fresh ingredients. The journey was about more than simply cooking; it was about regaining control of my body, listening to its messages and responding with care in the form of healthy food.

Imagine me as your culinary companion—a buddy in the kitchen, a guide on this gourmet adventure—while I share these dishes with you. Let us break bread together, savouring the flavour of fresh ingredients and revelling in the delight that comes from caring for our bodies.

The following pages are not merely a collection of recipes but also a road map to a healthier, more vibrant self. We'll dig into the art of making gut-friendly breakfasts that set the tone for the day, lunches that enrich the midday experience, and dinners that say goodbye to weariness. Snacks, sides, soups, salads, meat, poultry, and seafood are all woven into the fabric of a gut-healthy diet.

So, whether you're an experienced home cook or just starting, remember that this journey is about development, not perfection. It's about relishing preparing meals that love you back, one mouthful at a time.

Allow the fragrances, textures, and tastes to pique our interest and awe as we turn the pages together. The kitchen is more than simply a place to cook; it's a sanctuary where we grow energy, and I want you to make it your own with these recipes.

Gut Bliss is waiting for you—let the gastronomic experience begin!

Understanding Digestive Health

Understanding gut health is like interpreting the tremendous symphony playing within our bodies—a symphony orchestrated by billions of bacteria living in our digestive tract. The gut, sometimes known as the "second brain," is more than just a digestive organ; it is a dynamic ecosystem critical to our health.

The balance and variety of these bacteria, collectively known as the gut microbiome, is crucial to gut health. This complex ecosystem impacts everything from digestion and food absorption to immune function and mental health. A healthy gut microbiome is characterized by a diverse population of beneficial bacteria that strongly defend against infections and inflammation.

The microbiological fin link emphasizes the importance of gut health for mental and emotional balance. An unbalanced microbiome has been related to a variety of illnesses other than digestive issues, such as anxiety, depression, and autoimmune disorders.

Recognizing the symbiotic link between our lifestyle choices and this microbial universe is essential for understanding gut health. Nutrition, stress management, and mindful eating are all important. We support these bacteria to flourish by creating a gut-friendly environment with whole foods, prebiotics, and probiotics, resulting in a resilient and healthy gut.

Knowing gut health, in essence, goes beyond knowing digestion; it reveals the complex interaction between our food choices and the delicate microbial dance within, forming the cornerstone of our overall well-being.

The Importance of Gut Health

The significance of a healthy gut is inextricably linked to the transformational power of food. Aside from its role in digesting, the gut is an important factor in general health. Providing the correct meals to this critical ecosystem is analogous to developing a flourishing well-being garden.

A healthy gut is essential for nutrient absorption, ensuring that our food becomes an energy source for our whole body. It acts as a protector, boosting our immune system against intruders and encouraging strong resistance.

Furthermore, the gut-brain axis plays an important role in mood regulation. Nutrient-rich diets, particularly those high in prebiotics and probiotics, provide a harmonious habitat for beneficial bacteria, which positively impacts mental health. This inherent link emphasizes the importance of dietary choices on emotional balance and cognitive performance.

We can help our gut flora thrive by eating a diet high in fibre, different fruits and vegetables, fermented foods, and lean meats. These foods serve as allies, fostering a varied microbial community that improves digestion and adds to overall health. Thus, the significance of a healthy gut reverberates through our food choices, affecting how we fuel our bodies and laying the groundwork for long-term well-being.

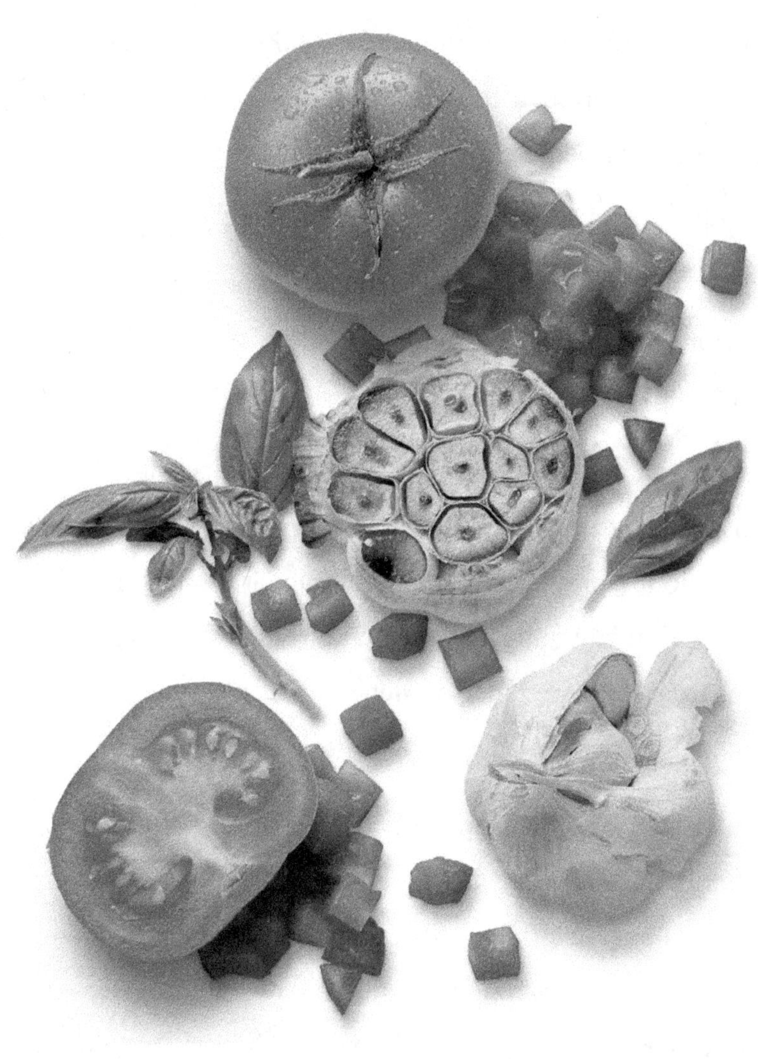

Chapter 1

Breakfast Delights

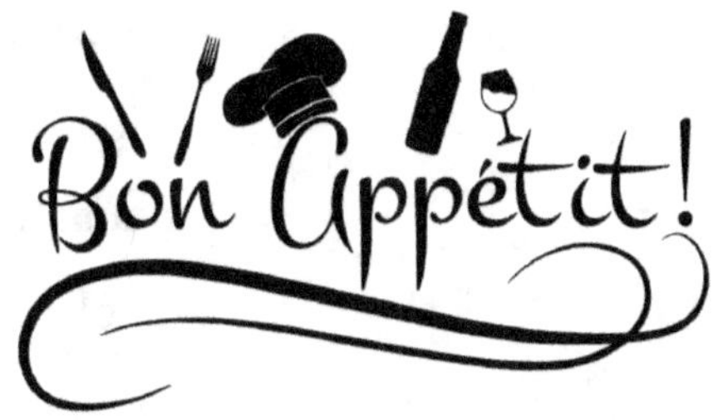

Breakfast Delights, chapter one, invites you to appreciate the morning routine with gut-friendly delicacies. Each meal, from vivid smoothie bowls to cozy overnight oats, is designed to feed your stomach and jumpstart a day of vigour. Breakfast becomes a moment of balance and wellness—a tasty precursor to a day of nutrition. Join us on this culinary adventure, where each mouthful is a step toward a healthy stomach and a productive day ahead.

Berry-Probiotic Smoothie Bowl ★★★★★

Ingredients:

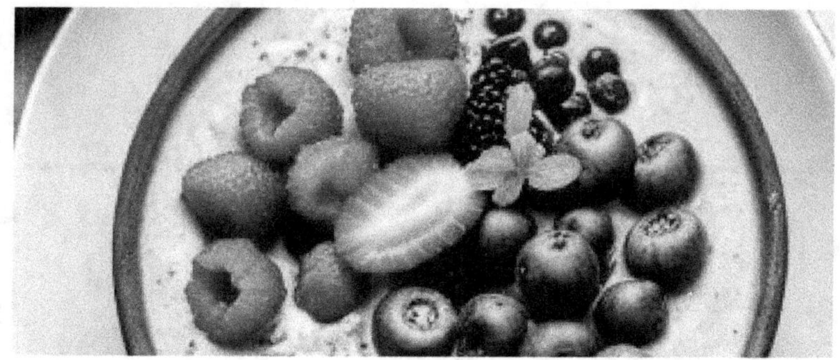

- 1 cup mixed berries (blueberries, strawberries, raspberries)
- 1/2 cup Greek yoghurt
- 1 banana ripe
- 1 teaspoon chia seeds
- Honey for drizzling (optional)
- Granola and fresh berries for topping

Preparation:

1. Blend the mixed berries, Greek yoghurt, banana, and chia seeds.
2. Blend until the mixture is smooth and creamy.
3. Transfer the smoothie to a bowl.

Toppings:

4. Top with a liberal sprinkling of granola for crunch.
5. Garnish with more berries if desired.
6. If preferred, drizzle with honey for added sweetness.

Nutritional Values (per Serving):

- 300 calories
- 15g protein
- 8g fibre
- 5g healthy fats

- 45g carbohydrates

Time to cook: 5 minutes

Oatmeal with Gut-Friendly See ★★★★★

Ingredients:

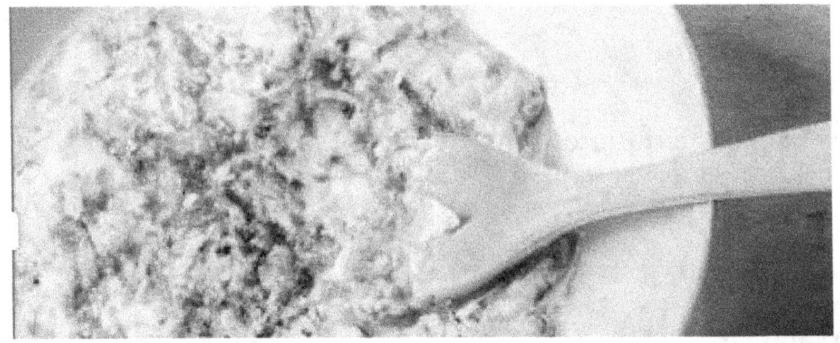

- 1/2 cup rolled oats
- 1/2 cup almond milk
- 1/2 cup Greek yogurt
- One teaspoon honey (optional)

- 1 tablespoon chia seeds
- 1 tablespoon flaxseeds
- 1 tablespoon pumpkin seeds
- Fresh berries for garnish

Preparation:

1. In a container, Combine the rolled oats, almond milk, Greek yoghurt, chia seeds, flaxseeds, and pumpkin seeds.
2. Stir thoroughly before sealing the container.
3. Place in the refrigerator overnight.

4. Mix the oats and sprinkle with honey, if preferred, in the morning.

5. Garnish with fresh berries.

Nutritional Values (per Serving):

- Calories: 320
- Protein: 15g
- Fiber: 10g
- Healthy Fats: 12g
- Carbohydrates: 35g

Time to cook: 5 minutes (plus overnight refrigerated)

Breakfast Muffins with Spinach and Feta

Ingredients:

★★★★★

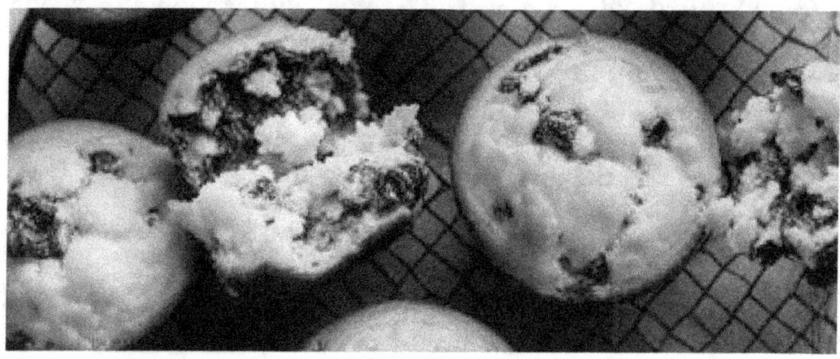

- 2 cups fresh spinach, chopped
- 1/2 cup feta cheese
- Crumbled 6 eggs
- 1/2 cup milk
- Salt and pepper to taste.
- Cooking spray or muffin liners

Preparation:

1. Heat the oven to 375°F (190°C).

2. Mix the eggs, milk, salt, and pepper in a dish.

3. Combine the egg mixture with the spinach and feta.

4. Spray or line a muffin pan with cooking spray.

5. Divide the mixture evenly among the muffin cups.

6. Bake the muffins for 20-25 minutes until they are firm and slightly brown.

Nutritional Values (per Muffin):

- Calories: 120
- Protein: 10g
- Healthy Fats: 7g
- Carbohydrates: 3g

Time to cook: 25 minutes

Parfait with Chia Seed Pudding ★★★★★

Ingredients:

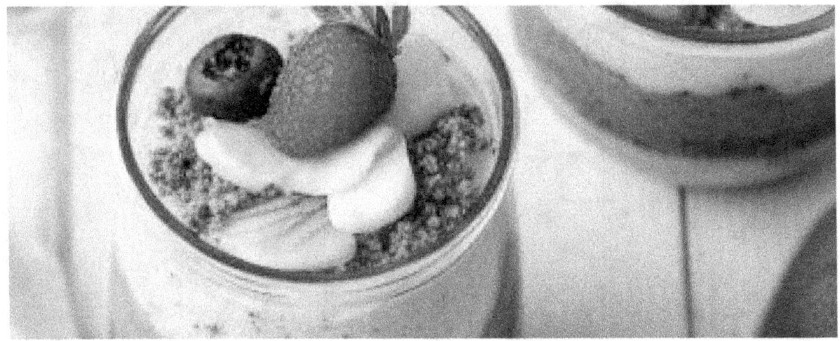

- 1/4 cup chia seeds
- 1 cup almond milk,
- 1 teaspoon vanilla extract

- 1 tablespoon maple syrup (optional)
- Greek yoghurt
- Fresh berries Granola

Preparation

1. In a container, Combine chia seeds, almond milk, vanilla essence, and maple syrup.
2. Stir thoroughly and place in the refrigerator for at least 2 hours or overnight until thickened.
3. Layer chia pudding, Greek yogurt, fresh berries, and granola in a glass.
4. Continue with the layers.

Nutritional Values (per Serving):

- Calories: 280
- Protein: 10g
- Fiber: 12g
- Healthy Fats: 8g
- Carbohydrates: 35g

Cooking Time: 5 minutes (plus cooling time

Breakfast Bowl with Quinoa ★★★★★

Ingredients:

- 1/2 cup cooked quinoa
- 1/2 cup almond milk
- Sliced almonds
- Fresh berries
- Maple syrup or honey
- Optional chia seeds

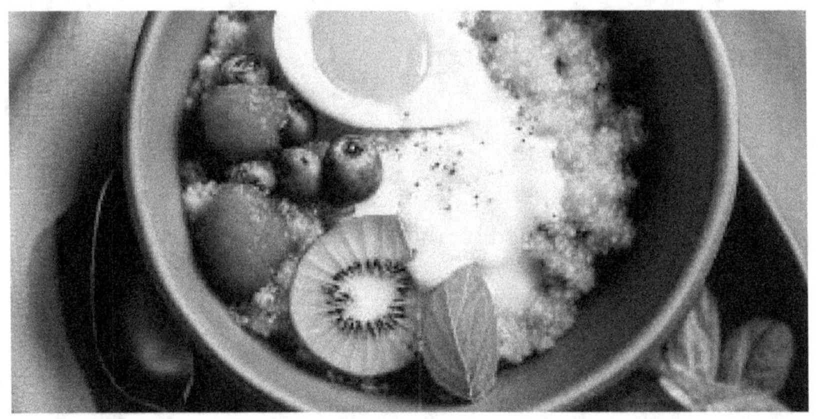

Preparation:

1. In a mixing dish, combine cooked quinoa and almond milk.

2. Garnish with sliced almonds, fresh berries, and maple syrup drizzle.

3. If preferred, add chia seeds.

Nutritional Values (per Serving):

- 300 calories
- 8g protein
- 7g fibre
- 10g healthy fats
- 45g carbohydrates

Cooking Time: 15 minutes (to prepare the quinoa)

Dear Health Advocates,

Prepare to be transformed by the transforming power of healthy, gut-loving meals. Our cookbook, is your entry point into a life where every food adds to your general well-being.

Consider a culinary journey in which each meal is a carefully crafted step toward a regenerated you—one who is full of unlimited energy, joy, and resilience. This compilation is more than simply a cookbook; it's a road map to a way of life that transforms your kitchen into a nourishing sanctuary.

Dive into a vivid world where the sizzle of the pan and tantalizing fragrances lead you to better health. Each meal represents a significant investment in your vitality. Today is the first step on your path to becoming a more vibrant, energetic, and empowered version of yourself.

Cheers to the wonders of food and the great trip that lies ahead!

Believe in your abilities,

Joan, Your Culinary Motivator

Chapter 2:

Delicious Lunch

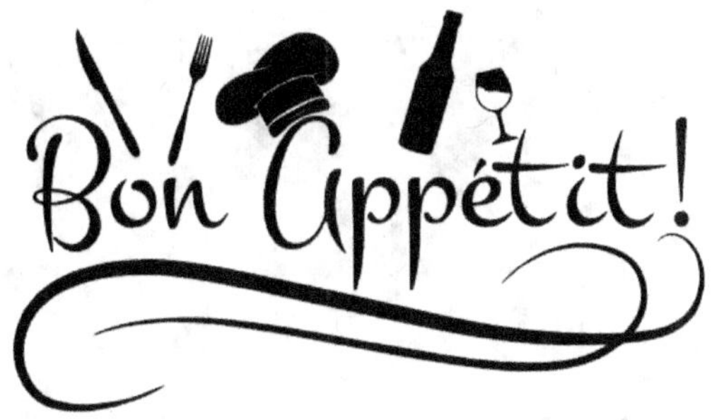

Enter the vivid world of "Lunch Unveiled," where midday meals are transformed into a feast of taste and health. In this chapter, we reimagine lunch, presenting a variety of recipes ranging from substantial bowls to protein-packed wraps that will boost your afternoon experience. Join us in the practice of mindful midday eating, where each cuisine is designed to satisfy your hunger and bring energy and vigor into your day. Lunch is no longer just a meal; it's an opportunity to experience gastronomic pleasures that nourish your body and spirit. Bon appétit!

Protein-Packed Lentil and Vegetable Wrap ★★★★★

Ingredients:

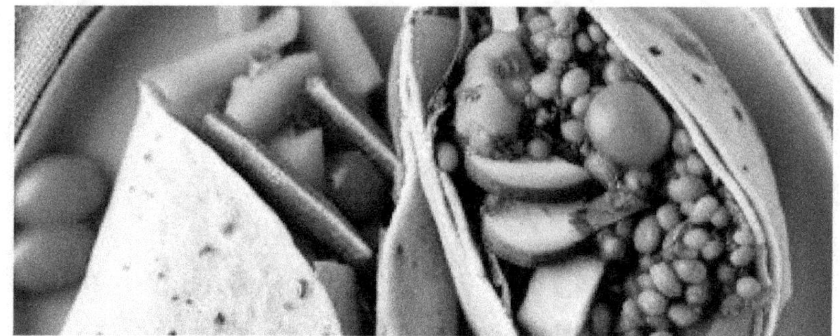

- 1 cup cooked lentils
- Whole-grain wraps
- Sliced mixed veggies (bell peppers, cucumbers, tomatoes)
- Hummus fresh greens (spinach or lettuce)
- Optional feta cheese
- Olive oil and lemon dressing

Preparation:

1. Spread hummus in the centre of a whole-grain wrap.
2. Stir in a heaping scoop of cooked lentils.
3. Arrange sliced mixed veggies and fresh greens on top.
4. Drizzle with the olive oil-lemon dressing.
5. Optional: Top with feta cheese.
6. Roll the wrap securely and cut it in half.

Nutritional Values (per wrap):

- 350 calories
- 18g protein
- 10g fibre
- 8g healthy fats
- 45g carbohydrates

Time to Cook: 15 minutes (for lentil preparation)

Salad with Quinoa and Fermented Veggies ★★★★★

Ingredients:

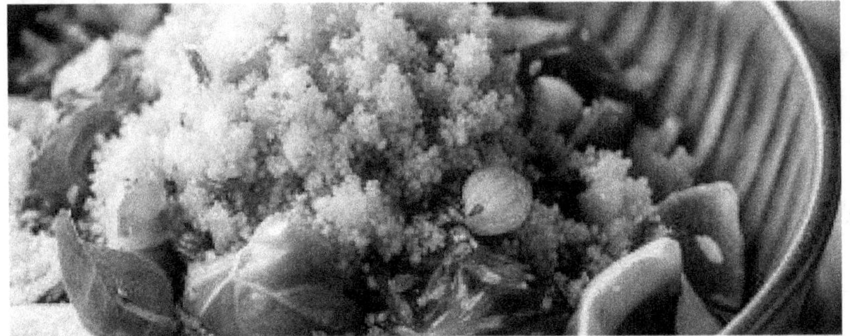

- 1 cup cooked quinoa
- Fermented vegetables (cabbage, carrots, radishes)
- Cherry tomatoes chopped
- Cucumber, diced
- Red onion thinly sliced
- Feta cheese, crumbled (optional)
- Dressing of fresh herbs (parsley or cilantro)
- Olive oil, and balsamic vinegar

Preparation:

1. Toss cooked quinoa with fermented vegetables, cherry tomatoes, cucumber, and red onion in a mixing dish.
2. If preferred, top with crumbled feta cheese.
3. Dress with olive oil and balsamic vinegar.
4. Garnish with fresh herbs.
5. Gently toss the salad until completely incorporated.

Nutritional Values (per Serving):

- Calories: 280
- Protein: 10g
- Fiber: 8g
- Healthy Fats: 10g
- 35g carbohydrates

Cooking Time: 15 minutes (to prepare the quinoa)

Chicken and Avocado Quinoa Bowl

Ingredients: ★★★★★

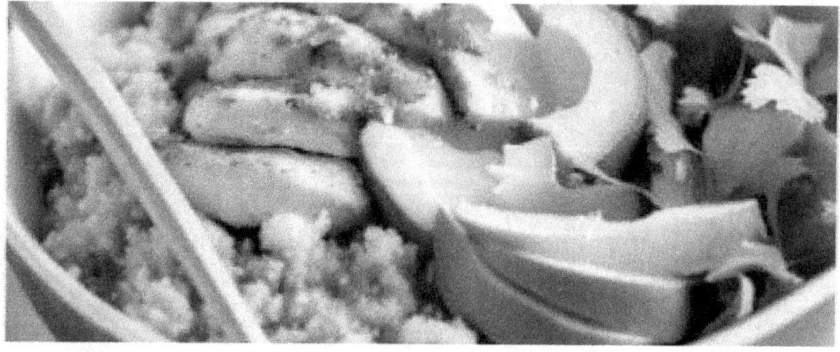

- 1 cup cooked quinoa
- Grilled chicken breast, sliced
- Avocado, sliced
- Cherry tomatoes, halved

- Black beans, drained and rinsed
- Corn kernels (fresh or canned)
- Cilantro, chopped
- Lime wedges
- Greek yogurt (optional, for topping)

Preparation:

1. Place the cooked quinoa in a mixing basin.
2. Arrange grilled chicken slices, avocado, cherry tomatoes, black beans, and corn on top.
3. Garnish with cilantro, if using.
4. Squeeze the lime wedges over the top of the bowl.
5. Optionally, top with a dollop of Greek yogurt.

Nutritional Values (per Serving):

- 400 calories
- 25g protein
- 12g fibre
- 15g healthy fats
- 45g carbohydrate

Cooking Time: 20 minutes (including preparation of the quinoa and chicken)

Mediterranean Chickpea Salad ★★★★★

Ingredients:

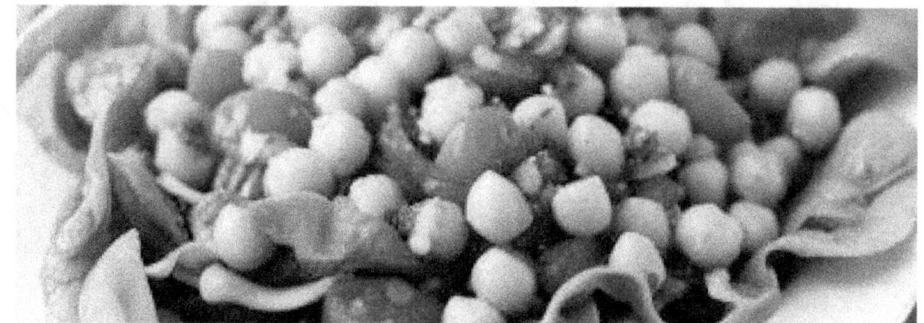

- 1 can (15 oz) chickpeas, drained and rinsed
- Cucumber, diced
- Cherry tomatoes, halved
- Kalamata olives, sliced
- Red onion, finely chopped
- Feta cheese, crumbled
- Fresh parsley, chopped
- Olive oil and lemon juice dressing
- Salt and pepper to taste

Preparation:

1. Combine chickpeas, diced cucumber, cherry tomatoes, olives, red onion, and crumbled feta in a mixing dish.
2. Drizzle with a mixture of olive oil and lemon juice.
3. Season with salt and pepper to taste.
4. Toss the salad until evenly combined.
5. Garnish with fresh parsley, if desired.

Nutritional Values (per Serving):

- 320 calories
- 12g protein
- 10g fibre
- 15g healthy fats
- 40g carbohydrates

Time to cook: 10 minutes (if using canned chickpeas)

Salad with Sweet Potatoes and Kale

Ingredients:

⭐⭐⭐⭐⭐

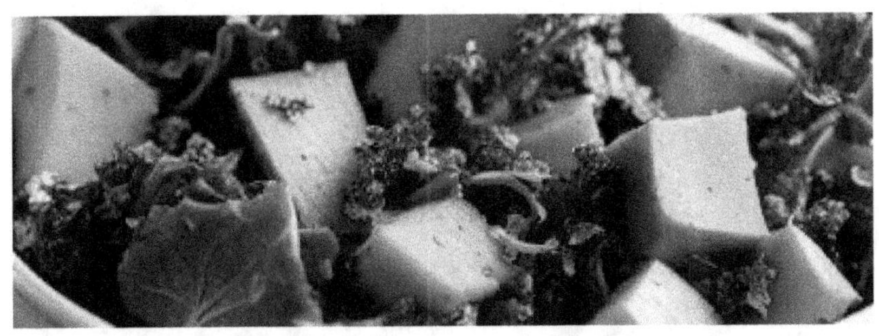

- Sweet potatoes, peeled and cubed
- Kale, stems removed and chopped
- Olive oil
- Maple syrup
- Pecans, chopped
- Dried cranberries
- Feta cheese, crumbled
- Balsamic vinaigrette

Preparation:

1. Toss sweet potato cubes with olive oil and maple syrup before roasting until soft.
2. To soften the kale, massage it with olive oil.
3. Toss together roasted sweet potatoes, kale, nuts, dried cranberries, and crumbled feta in a mixing dish.
4. Toss the salad with the balsamic vinaigrette.

Nutritional Values (per Serving):

- 350 calories
- 8g protein
- 10g fibre
- 15g healthy fats
- 45g carbohydrates

Time to cook: 25 minutes (including cooking sweet potatoes)

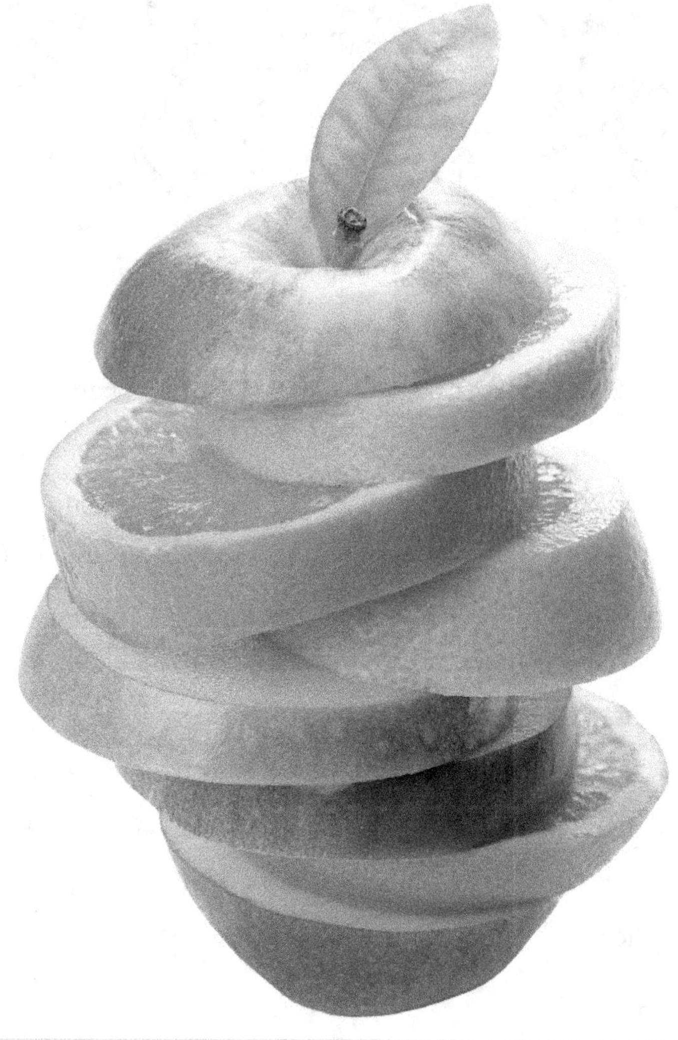

Chapter 3:

Dinner Harmony

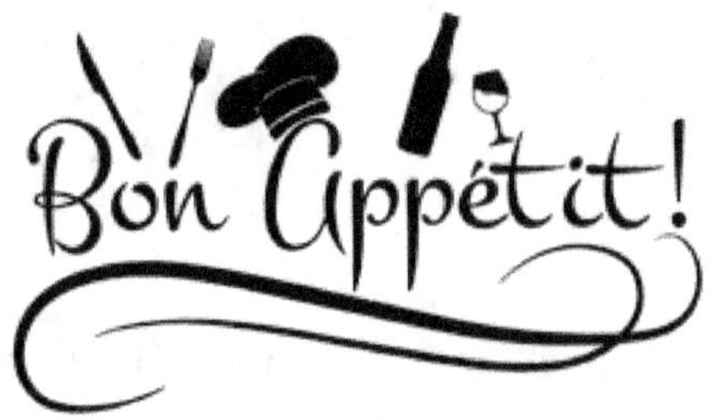

As the sun sets, we enter the enchanted world of "Dinner Harmony." This chapter weaves a tapestry of evening meals meant to transcend the mundane and provide more than simply nutrition but a symphony of flavours and nutrients. Dinner is a celebration on this culinary journey—a chance to appreciate healthful foods that end the day positively.

Salmon Baked with Lemon and Dill

Ingredients: ★★★★★

- Salmon fillets
- Fresh lemon slices

- Chopped fresh dill
- Olive oil
- Garlic powder
- Salt and pepper to taste

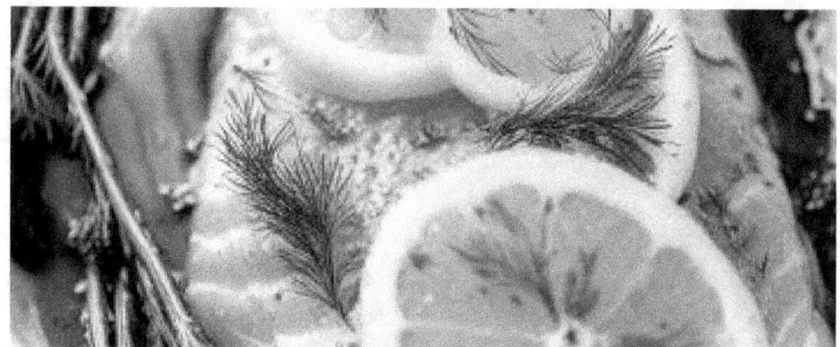

Preparation:

1. Preheat the oven to 375 degrees Fahrenheit (190 degrees Celsius).
2. Place the salmon fillets on a baking sheet with parchment paper.
3. Drizzle with olive oil and season with garlic powder, salt, and pepper to taste.
4. Garnish each fillet with fresh lemon slices and dill.
5. Bake for 15-20 minutes or until the fish is well cooked.

Nutritional Values (per Serving):

- Calories: 300
- Protein: 25g
- Healthy Fats: 18g
- Carbohydrates: 2g

Time to cook: 20 minutes

Veggie Stir-Fry Tofu ★★★★★

Ingredients:

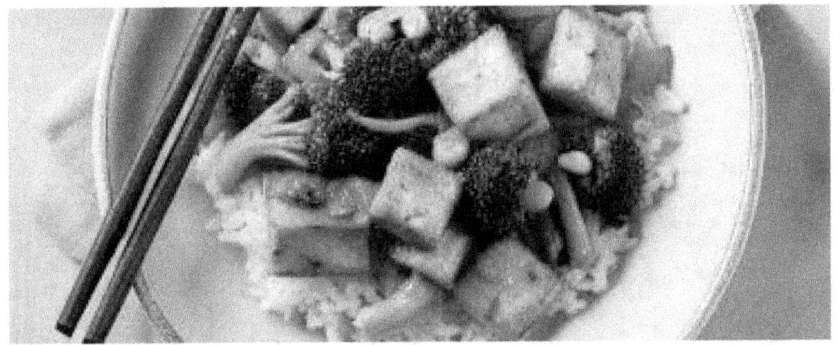

- Firm tofu, cubed
- Mixed veggies (bell peppers, broccoli, carrots, snap peas), sliced Soy sauce
- Sesame seed oil
- Sliced green onions
- Grated garlic
- Minced ginger
- Optional sesame seeds

Preparation:

1. Remove extra water from tofu and cut into cubes.
2. Sauté tofu in sesame oil in a wok or pan until brown.
3. Stir in the minced garlic and grated ginger until fragrant.
4. Add the mixed veggies and continue to stir-fry until crisp-tender.
5. Toss with the soy sauce to mix.
6. If preferred, garnish with sliced green onions and sesame seeds.

Nutritional Values (per Serving):

- Calories: 250
- Protein: 18g

- Healthy Fats: 12g
- Carbohydrates: 15g

Time to cook: 15 minutes

Turmeric-Ginger Chicken Skewers

Ingredients: ★★★★★

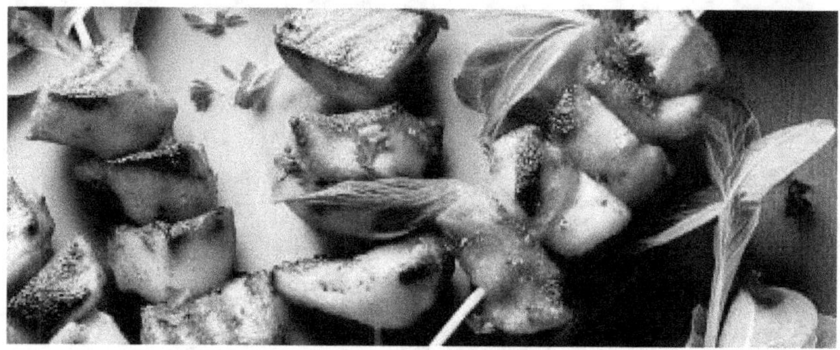

- Chicken breast, cubed
- Turmeric powder
- Fresh ginger
- Grated garlic
- Minced Yogurt
- Lemon juice
- Olive oil
- Salt and pepper to taste

Preparation:

1. add yoghurt, turmeric powder, grated ginger, minced garlic, lemon juice, olive oil, salt, and pepper in a mixing bowl to make a marinade.

2. Thread the chicken cubes onto skewers and cover them thoroughly in the marinade.

3. Marinate for at least 30 minutes or overnight in the refrigerator.

4. Preheat the grill or oven to high heat.

5. Grill or bake the skewers until the chicken is brown.

Nutritional Values (per Serving):

- Calories: 280
- Protein: 25g
- Healthy Fats: 10g
- Carbohydrates: 15g

Time to cook: 15-20 minutes (including marination and cooking)

Stuffed Peppers with Quinoa and Black Beans ★★★★★

Ingredients:

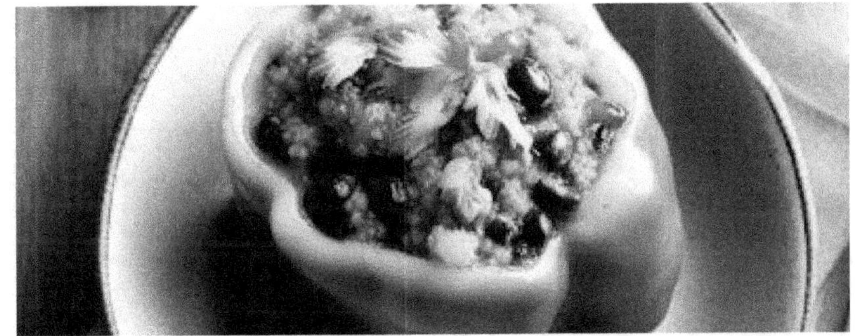

- Bell peppers, halved and seeds removed
- Cooked quinoa
- Black beans washed and rinsed
- Corn kernels (fresh or frozen)
- Salsa Cumin powder
- Chilli powder
- Shredded cheese (cheddar or Mexican blend)

- Chopped fresh cilantro (for garnish)

Preparation:

1. Preheat the oven to 375 degrees Fahrenheit (190 degrees Celsius).
2. Combine cooked quinoa, black beans, corn, salsa, cumin powder, and chilli powder in a mixing bowl.
3. Stuff each bell pepper half with the quinoa and black bean mixture.
4. Garnish with shredded cheese.
5. Bake for 20-25 minutes until the peppers are soft and the cheese has melted.
6. Before serving, garnish with fresh cilantro.

Nutritional Values (per Serving):

- 300 calories
- 12g protein
- 8g fibre
- 8g healthy fats
- 45g carbohydrates

Time to cook: 25 minutes

Brown Rice Pilaf with Mixed Vegetables

Ingredients: ★★★★★

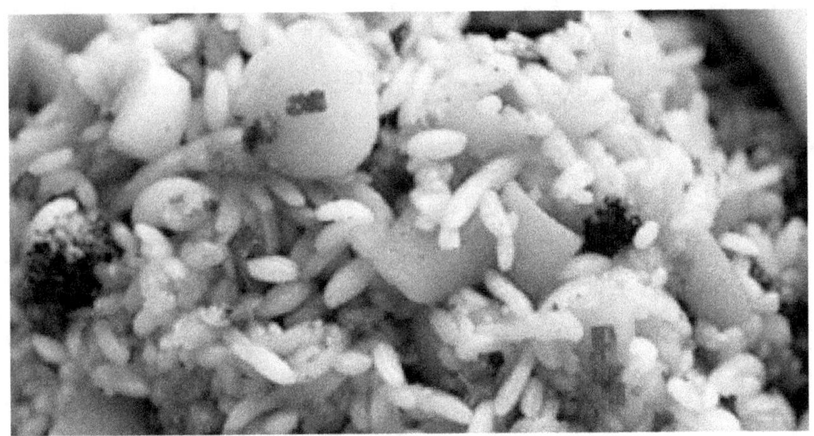

- Brown rice
- Mixed vegetables (carrots, peas, corn)
- Onion, finely chopped
- Garlic, minced
- Vegetable broth
- Olive oil
- Fresh parsley, chopped (for garnish)
- Salt and pepper to taste

Preparation:

1. Sauté chopped onion and garlic in olive oil in a saucepan until softened.
2. Stir in the brown rice to coat it with the oil.
3. Bring the vegetable broth to a boil.
4. Reduce heat to low, cover, and simmer until rice is tender and liquid has been absorbed.
5. Add mixed veggies in the last 10 minutes of boiling and continue to simmer until tender.

6. Fluff the rice with a fork and season it with salt and pepper before garnishing it with fresh parsley.

Nutritional Values (per Serving):

- Calories: 220
- Protein: 5g
- Fiber: 6g
- Healthy Fats: 4g
- 40g carbohydrates

Cooking Time: 45 minutes (including cooking time for the vegetables)

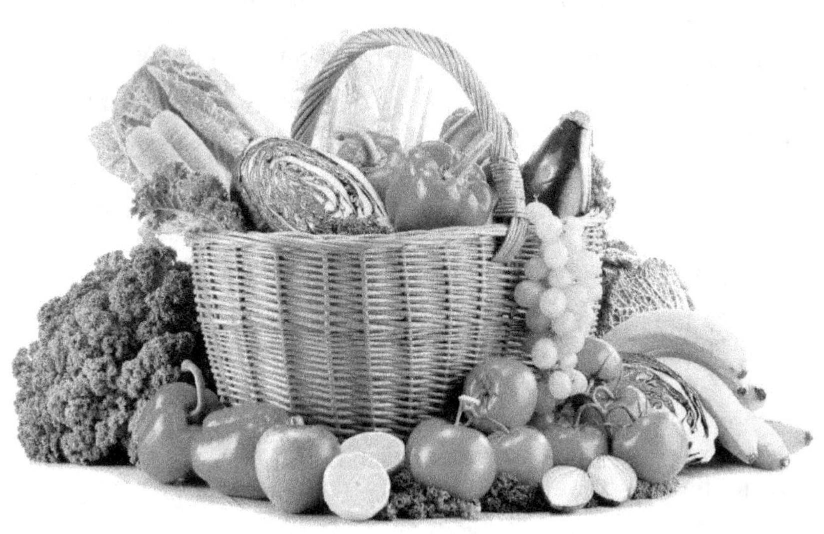

Chapter 4.

Savoring Snacks

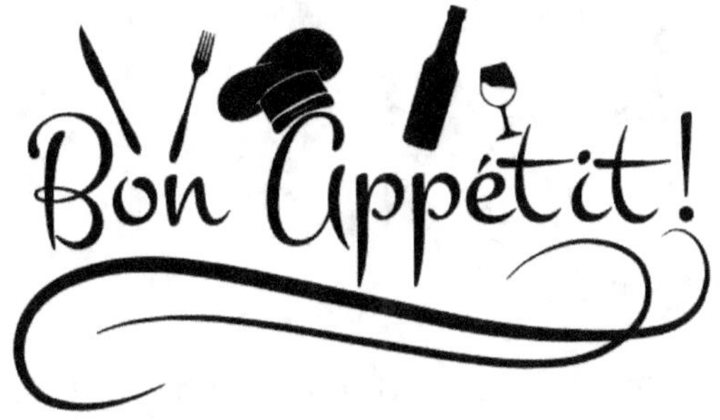

Savoring Moments urges you to indulge in snacks that go beyond nourishment while we travel between meals. This chapter is dedicated to the tasty morsels that offer a symphony of flavors and a burst of energy to your day. Each dish, from guilt-free nibbles to savory delights, is intended to convert snack time into a sheer joy. Snack with gusto!

Parfait of Greek Yogurt with Berries and Granola ★★★★★

Ingredients:

- Yogurt from Greece

- Strawberries, blueberries, and raspberries • Granola
- Optional honey

- Mint leaves, fresh (for garnish)

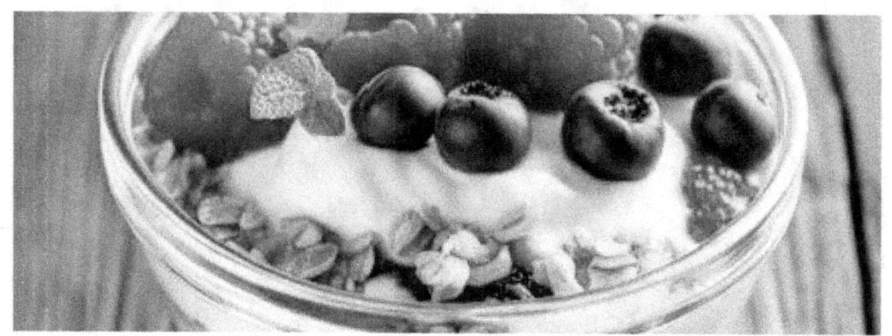

Preparation:

1. Cover the bottom of a glass or plate with Greek yogurt.
2. Add a layer of mixed berries on top.
3. Top with a thick layer of Granola.
4. Continue stacking until the container is completely filled.
5. Drizzle with honey if desired.
6. If preferred, garnish with fresh mint leaves.

Nutritional Information (per serving):

- 250 calories
- 15g protein
- 5g fiber

- 8g of good fats
- 35g carbohydrate

Cooking time: 5 minutes (assembly)

Spiced Roasted Chickpeas ★★★★★

Ingredients:

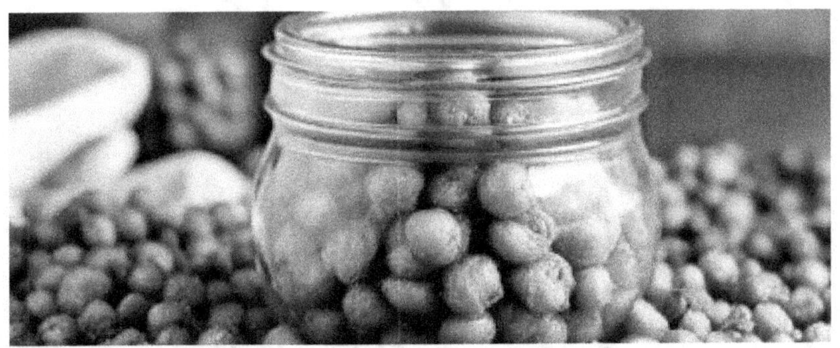

- Rinsed and Drained Canned Chickpeas
- olive oil
- smoked paprika
- cumin roasted garlic powder
- Salt and pepper

Preparation:

1. Preheat the oven to 400 degrees F (200 degrees C).
2. Pat dry the chickpeas with a paper towel to remove excess moisture.
3. In a mixing bowl, combine chickpeas, olive oil, smoked paprika, cumin, garlic powder, salt, and pepper.
4. Arrange the chickpeas on a baking sheet in a single layer.
5. Roast for 25-30 minutes, or until crispy, stirring halfway through.

Nutritional Information (per serving):

- 180 calories
- 7g protein
- 5g fiber
- 6g healthy fats
- 25g carbohydrates

Cooking time of 30 minutes

Nut and Seed Trail Mix ★★★★★

Ingredients.

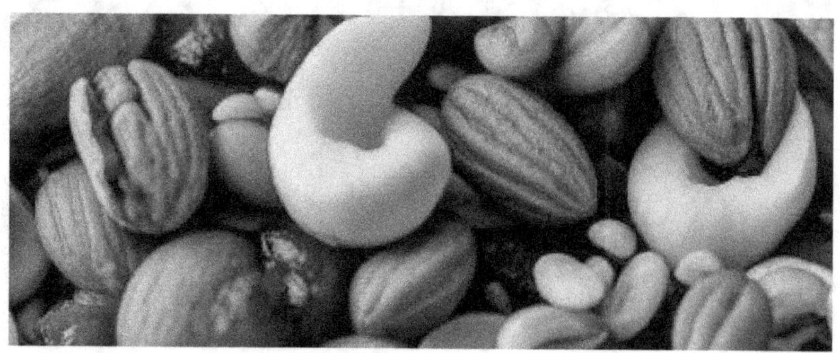

- Almond, walnuts, pumpkin seeds, sunflower seeds, dried cranberries
- Dark chocolate chips

Preparation:

1. In a mixing bowl, blend almonds, walnuts, pumpkin seeds, sunflower seeds, dried cranberries, and dark chocolate chips.
2. Toss until well blended.

Nutritional Information (per serving):

- 200 calories
- 8g protein • 4g fiber

- Carbohydrates: 15g
- Healthy Fats: 15g

Cooking time: 5 minutes (assembly)

Hummus on Veggie Sticks 

Ingredients:

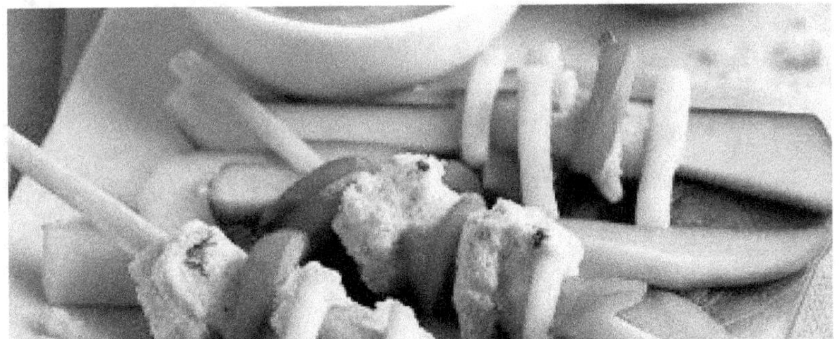

- Hummus (either store-bought or homemade)
- Carrot sticks
- Cucumber slices
- Bell pepper strips

Preparation:

1. Place carrot sticks, cucumber slices, and bell pepper strips on a serving plate.
2. Serve with a serving of hummus for dipping.

Nutritional Values (per Serving):

- Calories: 150
- Protein: 5g • 8g fiber
- 10g of healthy fats
- 15g of carbohydrates

Cooking time: 5 minutes (assembly)

Almond Butter Apple Slices ★★★★★

Ingredients:

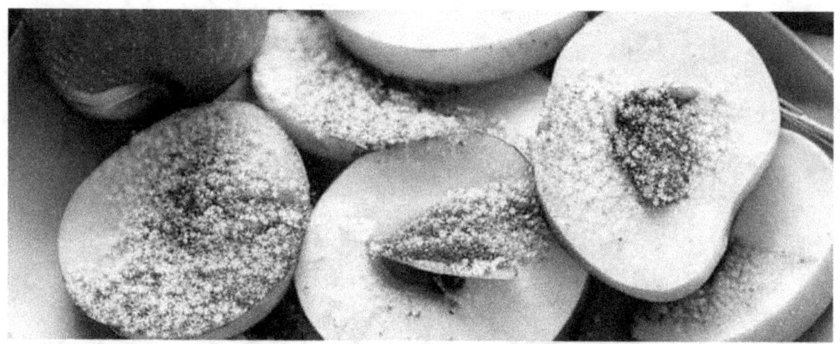

- Sliced apples
- Almond butter

Preparation:

1. Peel and cut the apples into wedges.

2. Spread a thin coating of almond butter on each apple slice.

Nutritional data (per serving):

- 180 calories
- Healthy Fats: 10g
- Protein: 3g
- Carbohydrates: 20g
- Fiber: 5g

Cooking time: 5 minutes (assembly)

Chapter 5:

A Delicious Side Dish

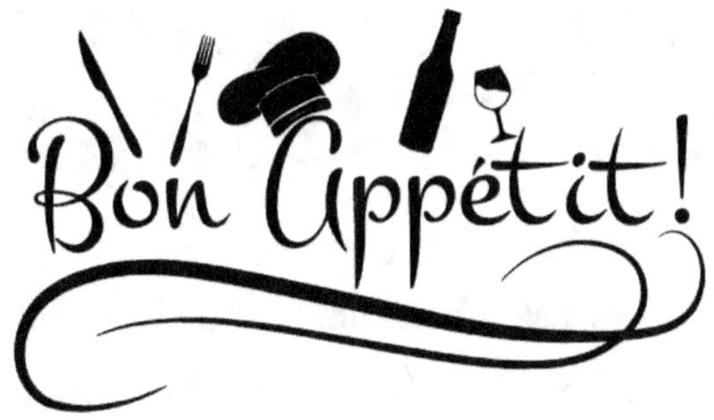

Side dishes are the unsung heroes of the kitchen, lifting a meal from ordinary to exceptional. "Good Side Dish" transports you to a world where these culinary companions take center stage. This chapter is dedicated to the art of side dishes, from vibrant salads that cleanse the palate to hearty grains that complement the main course.

Let the delectable symphony begin!

Fermented Cabbage Slaw ★★★★★

Ingredients:

- Thinly sliced cabbage
- Grated carrots
- Sea salt
- Caraway seeds

- (Optional) berries of juniper

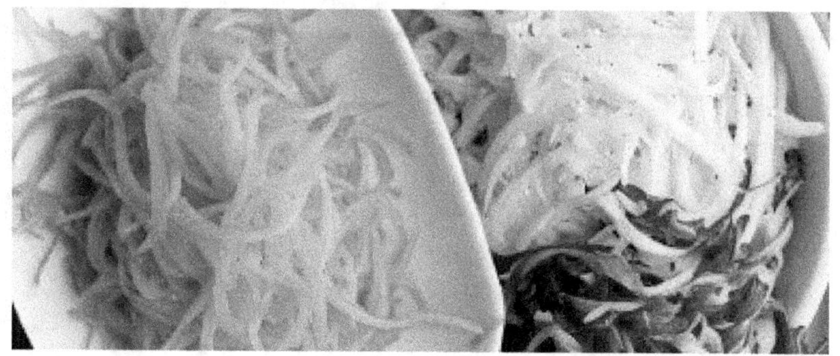

Preparation:

1. In a mixing bowl, combine shredded cabbage and grated carrots.

2. Season the vegetables with sea salt and knead until liquid is released.

3. Submerge the mixture entirely in its liquid in a jar.

4. Fold in the juniper berries and caraway seeds.

5. Cover the jar and set it aside at room temperature to ferment for 1-2 weeks.

Nutritional Values (per Serving):

- 30 Calories
- 4g Fiber
- 30% DV Vitamin C
- Probiotics for intestinal health

Cooking/fermentation time: 1-2 weeks (fermentation).

Sweet Potatoes Roasted with Garlic and Herbs ★★★★★

Ingredients:

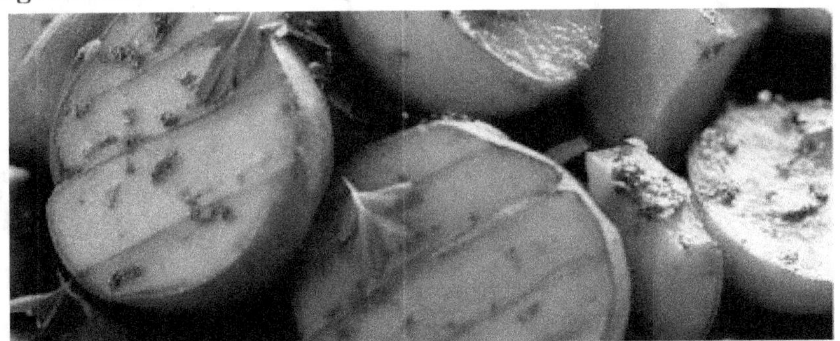

- Sweet potatoes, peeled and cubed
- Olive oil
- Garlic, minced
- Fresh herbs (rosemary or thyme), chopped
- Salt and pepper to taste

Preparation:

1. Preheat the oven to 400 degrees F (200 degrees C).
2. Combine the cubed sweet potatoes, olive oil, garlic, fresh herbs, salt, and pepper in a mixing bowl.
3. Arrange the sweet potatoes on a baking sheet in a single layer.
4. Bake for approximately 25-30 minutes, or until golden brown and tender.

Nutritional Values (per Serving):

- 150 calories
- 4g fiber

- 400% DV vitamin A
- 30% DV vitamin C

Cooking time of 30 minutes

Salad with Quinoa and Black Beans

Ingredients: ★★★★★

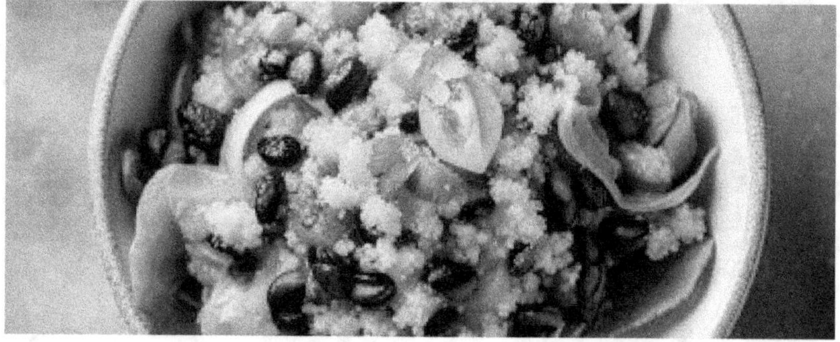

- Quinoa Black beans, tinned, drained, and rinsed
- Corn kernels (fresh or frozen)
- Halved cherry tomatoes
- Red onion, finely chopped
- Cilantro, chopped
- Lime juice
- Olive oil
- Salt and pepper to taste

Preparation:

1. Prepare the quinoa according to the package recommendations.
2. In a mixing bowl, combine cooked quinoa, black beans, corn, cherry tomatoes, red onion, and cilantro.
3. Drizzle with olive oil and lime juice to finish.
4. Season to taste with salt and pepper.
5. Gently mix the salad until well combined.

Nutritional Information (per Serving):

- 250 calories
- 10g protein
- 8g fiber
- 8g healthy fats
- 40g carbohydrates

Cooking time: 15 minutes (quinoa preparation).

Turmeric Cauliflower Mash ★★★★★

Ingredients:

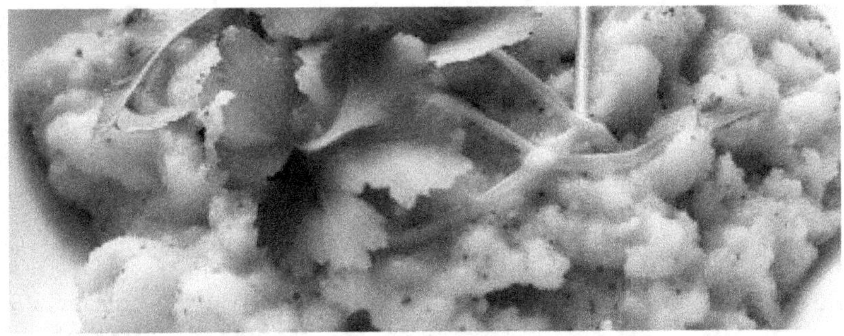

- Cauliflower florets
- Olive oil
- Turmeric powder
- Sliced garlic
- Salt & pepper to taste
- Fresh chopped parsley (optional)

Preparation:

1. Cook or steam the cauliflower until it is tender.

2. Mash the cauliflower with a fork or a potato masher.

3. In a pan, sauté minced garlic in olive oil until aromatic.

4. In a mixing dish, combine the mashed cauliflower, turmeric powder, salt, and pepper.

5. Stir completely and continue to cook for another 2-3 minutes.

6. Garnish with fresh parsley if desired.

Nutritional Information (per serving):

- 80g calories
- 5g fiber
- 70%DV vitamin C

- Turmeric contains anti-inflammatory properties.

Cooking time: 15 minutes

Greens Sautéed with Lemon and Pine Nuts ★★★★★

Ingredients:

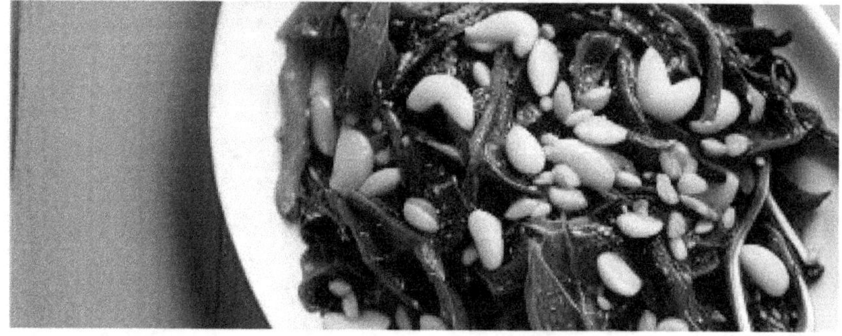

- Chopped mixed greens (kale, spinach, Swiss chard)
- Olive oil

- Minced garlic
- Lemon zest
- Pine nuts
- Salt and pepper to taste

Preparation:

1. In a pan, heat the olive oil and sauté the minced garlic until golden.

2. Add the chopped mixed greens and cook until wilted.

3. Combine the lemon zest and pine nuts in a mixing bowl.

4. Season to taste with salt and pepper.

5. Continue to cook for another 2-3 minutes.

Nutritional Information (per Serving):

- 120 calories
- 4g protein; 3g fiber; 9g healthy fats
- Vitamin A: 80% of the DV
- Vitamin C (40 DV)

Cooking time: 10 minutes

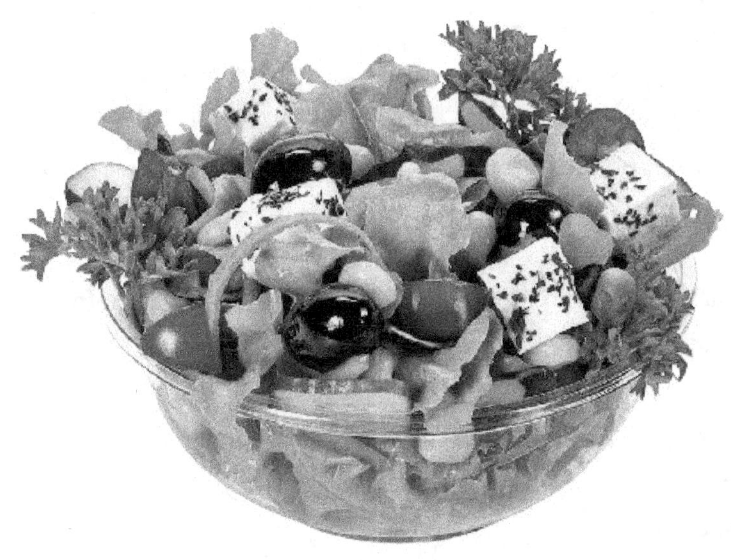

Dear Wellness Fighters,

Through the power of mindful nutrition, go on a transforming path to a healthier self. Your cookbook is more than simply a collection of recipes; it is also your road map to health.

Each dish is a step toward a more powerful, resilient self. Accept the power of mindful eating, where every item is a nutrient-dense ally on your wellness journey.

This isn't just about food; it's a way of life that embraces the symbiotic relationship between your decisions and the harmony of your body. You carve a masterpiece of energy with each mouthful.

Even if difficulties emerge, use them as stepping stones to victory. You are not just fueling your body, but also the roots of your power.

To a life driven by the highest quality ingredients, both in your kitchen and within yourself.

With my support,

Joan.

Chapter 6

Soups

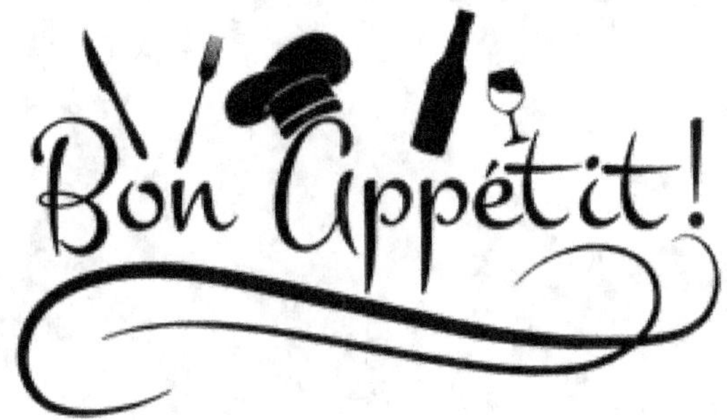

Simmering Comfort: Soups is a chapter dedicated to the warmth and comfort of a bowl. In this culinary adventure, we will learn how to make healthy soups that comfort the spirit and excite the taste senses. This chapter is a monument to the flexibility and richness of soups, with comforting stews that recall memories of home and vivid broths that energize the senses.

Enjoy the soothing taste of symphony!

Gut-Healing Bone Broth Soup ★★★★★

Ingredients:

- Chicken or cow bones
- Water
- Carrots, chopped
- Celery, chopped
- Onion, chopped
- Garlic, minced
- Fresh ginger, sliced
- Apple cider vinegar
- Salt and pepper to taste
- Chopped fresh parsley (for garnish)

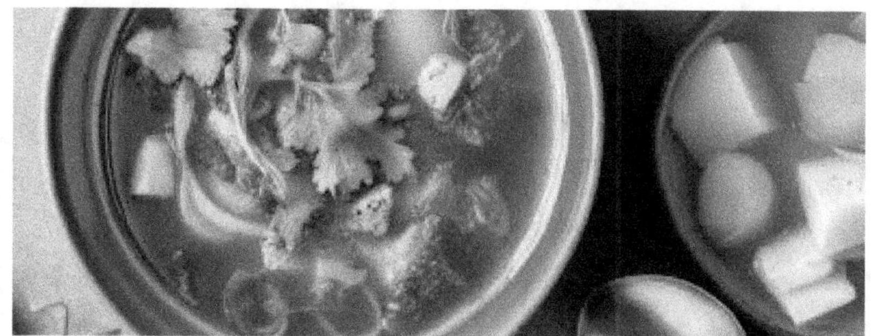

Preparation:

1. Place the bones in a big saucepan with water and apple cider vinegar. Allow it to settle for 30 minutes.
2. add the chopped veggies, Garlic, ginger, turmeric, Salt, and pepper to the saucepan.
3. Bring to a boil, then reduce to a low heat for 4 to 24 hours.
4. Strain the broth, discarding the particles but keeping the liquid.
5. Reheat, if necessary, then sprinkle with fresh parsley and serve.

Nutritional Values (per Serving):

- 40 calories
- 5g protein
- collagen for intestinal health

- essential minerals

Time to cook: 4-24 hours (simmering)

Creamy Butternut Squash Soup

Ingredients:

★★★★★

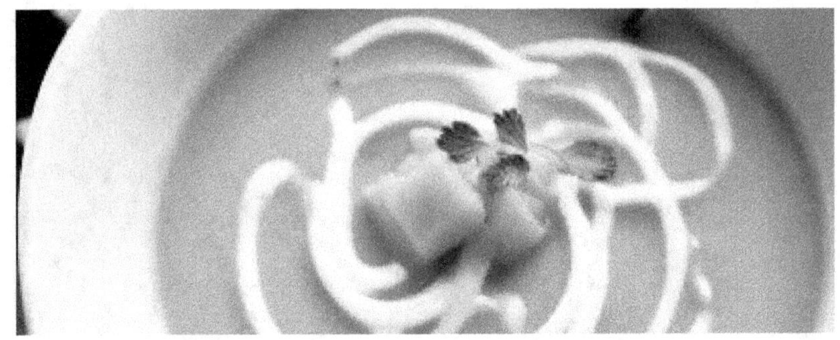

- Peeled and cubed butternut squash
- Chopped onion
- Chopped carrots
- Vegetable broth
- Coconut milk
- Nutmeg
- Salt and pepper to taste

Preparation:

1. In a skillet, sauté chopped Onion in olive oil until transparent.
2. Cook for 5 minutes after adding the diced butternut squash and carrots.
3. Pour the vegetable broth, boil, and then reduce to low heat until the veggies are cooked.
4. Puree the soup until smooth, then add the coconut milk and mix well.

5. Season with nutmeg, Salt, and pepper to taste.

Nutritional Values (per Serving):

- 150 Calories
- 5g fiber

- 300% DV vitamin A
- 40% DV vitamin C

Time to cook: 30 minutes

Soup with Whole Grains Minestrone

Ingredients:

★★★★★

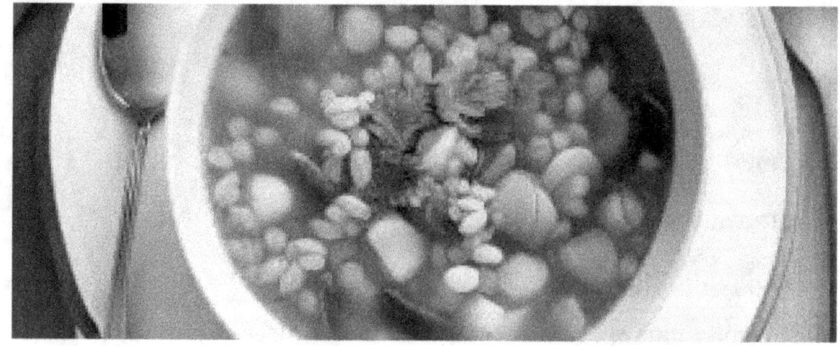

- Onion, diced
- Garlic, minced
- Carrots, sliced
- Celery, chopped
- Zucchini, diced
- Vegetable broth
- Cannellini beans, drained and rinsed

- Whole-grain pasta
- Fresh basil, chopped
- Olive oil
- Salt and pepper to taste
- Grated Parmesan cheese (optional for topping)

Preparation:

1. Cook the chopped Onion and Garlic in olive oil until softened.
2. In the oven, Stir in the cut carrots, celery, and cubed zucchini for 5 minutes.
3. Add the veggie broth and diced canned tomatoes. Bring to a boil.
4. Stir in whole-wheat pasta and cannellini beans. Cook the pasta until it is al dente.
5. Season with Salt, pepper, and fresh basil to taste.
6. Serve hot, topped with grated Parmesan cheese if desired.

Nutritional Information (per Serving):

- 250 calories
- 10g protein
- 8g fiber
- 5g healthy fats
- 45g carbohydrates

Time to cook: 30 minutes

Turmeric-Spiced Lentil Soup ★★★★★

Ingredients:

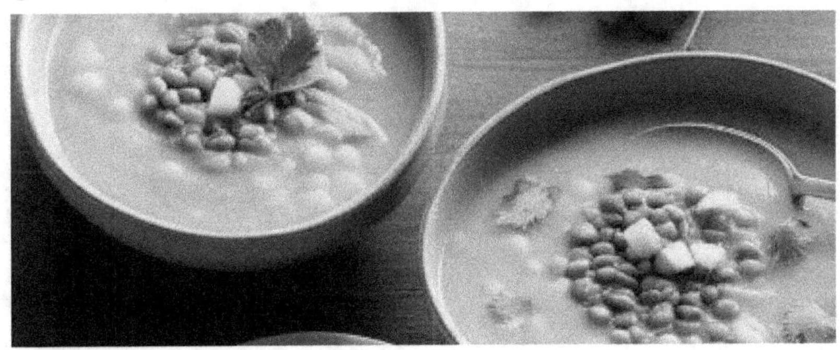

- Washed red lentils
- Chopped onion

- Minced garlic
- Sliced carrots
- Vegetable broth
- Ground turmeric
- Cumin powder
- Red pepper flakes (to taste)
- Olive oil
- Salt and pepper to taste
- Chopped fresh cilantro (for garnish)

Preparation:

1. In olive oil, sauté the chopped Onion and minced Garlic until aromatic.
2. Stir in the carrots and red lentils. 5 minutes in the oven.
3. To taste, Add vegetable broth, powdered turmeric, cumin powder, red pepper flakes, Salt, and pepper.
4. Bring to a boil, then reduce to low heat and cook until the lentils are cooked.
5. Before serving, garnish with fresh cilantro.

Nutritional Information (per Serving):

- 220 calories
- 12g protein
- 8g fiber
- 5g healthy fats
- 30g carbohydrates

Time to cook: 25 minutes

Chicken and Vegetable Quinoa Soup

Ingredients:

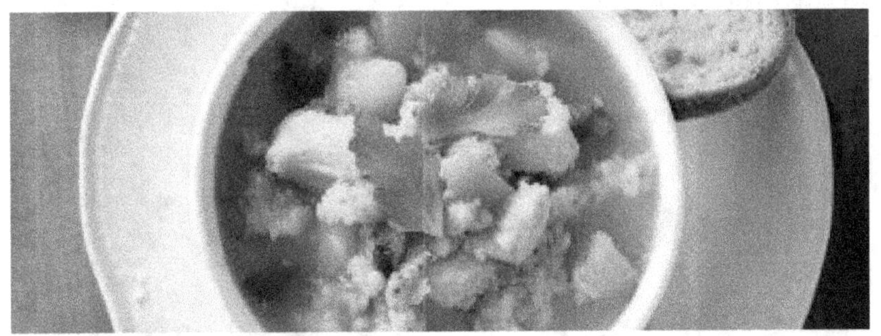

- Cooked and shredded chicken breast
- Washed quinoa
- Carrots, sliced
- Celery, chopped
- Onion, diced
- Garlic, minced
- Chicken broth
- Thyme
- Bay leaves
- Salt and pepper to taste

Preparation:

1. Sauté diced Onion and minced Garlic in a saucepan until tender.
2. Stir in the cut carrots, celery, shredded chicken, and rinsed quinoa. 5 minutes in the oven.
3. Season the chicken broth with thyme, bay leaves, Salt, and pepper.
4. Bring to a boil, then reduce to low heat and cook until the quinoa is soft and the veggies are tender.
5. Remove bay leaves and serve with fresh parsley.

Nutritional Values (per Serving):

- 300 calories
- 20g protein
- 5g fiber
- 5g healthy fats
- 40g carbohydrates

Time to cook: 30 minutes

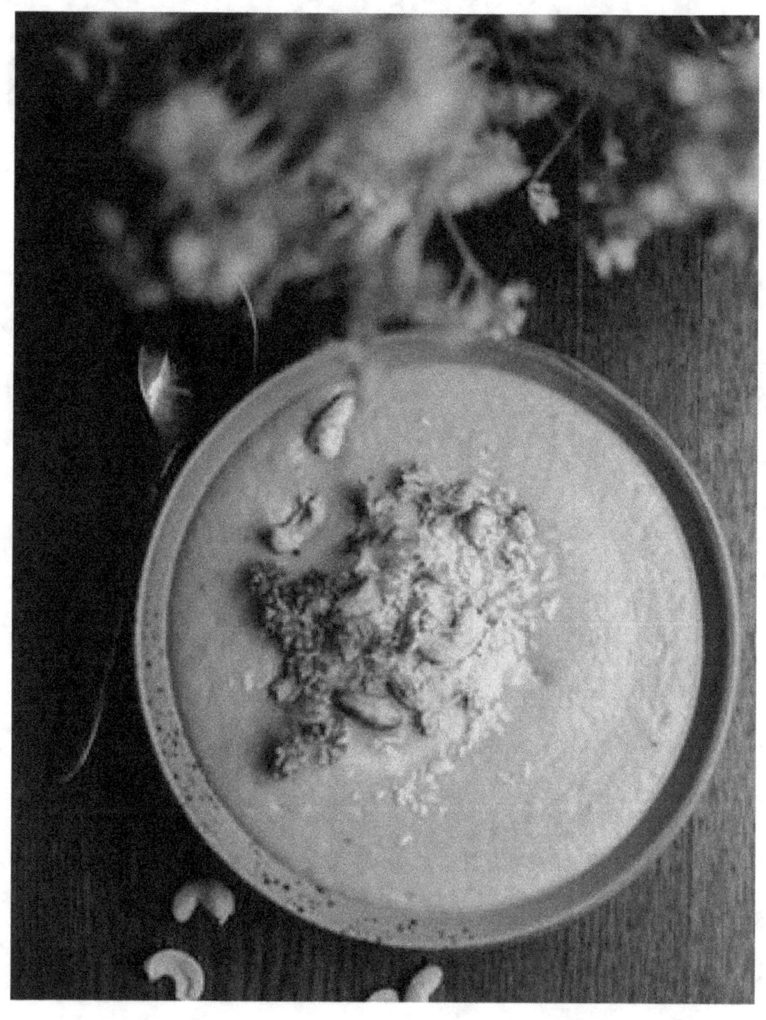

Chapter 7:

Salads

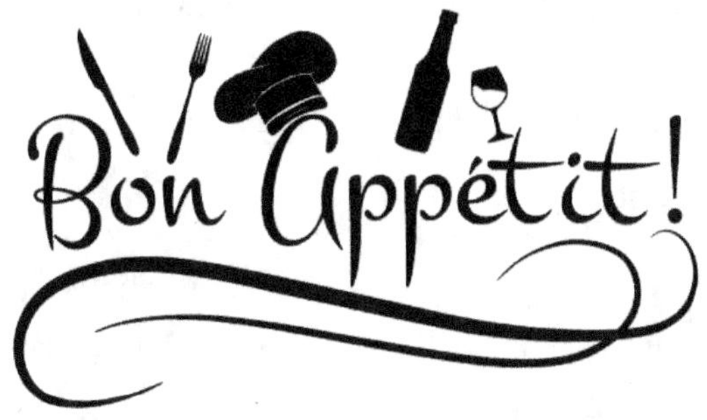

In the magnificent tapestry of "Harmony in Every Bite," our culinary adventure culminates with "Crisp Harmony: Salads." This chapter honors the culinary creativity in every salad dish, where freshness, brilliant colors, and nutritious ingredients take center stage. These salads are more than just side dishes; they celebrate nutrition, flavor, and the delight of clean dining.

Enjoy nature's brilliance, one salad at a time!

Salad with Avocado and Kale with Lemon Dressing ★★★★★

Ingredients:

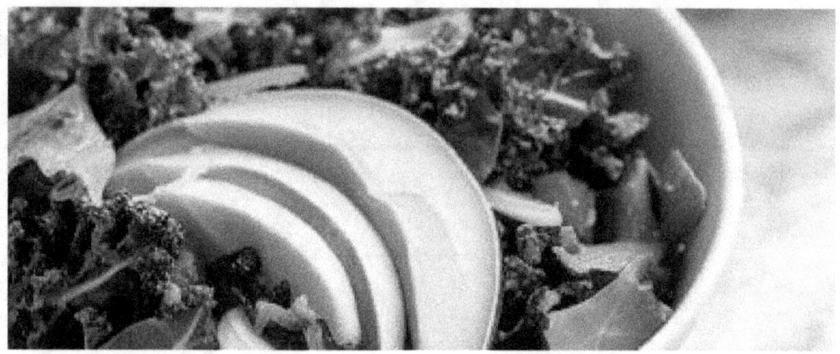

- Kale (stems removed and leaves chopped)
- Avocado (sliced)
- Cherry tomatoes (halved)
- Red onion (thinly sliced)
- Pumpkin seeds (optional)
- Olive oil
- Seasoning to taste
- Grated Parmesan cheese (optional, for garnish)

Preparation:

1. To soften the kale, rub it with lemon juice and olive oil in a large mixing bowl for 2-3 minutes.
2. Top with sliced avocado, cherry tomatoes, red Onion, and pumpkin seeds.
3. Toss the salad until everything is properly blended.
4. Season with Salt and pepper to taste.
5. If preferred, garnish with grated Parmesan cheese.

Nutritional Information (per Serving):

- 250 calories
- 7g protein
- 8g fiber
- 18g healthy fats

- 20g carbohydrates

Time to Cook: 10 minutes (preparation)

Beet and Walnut Salad with Apple Cider Vinaigrette ★★★★★

Ingredients:

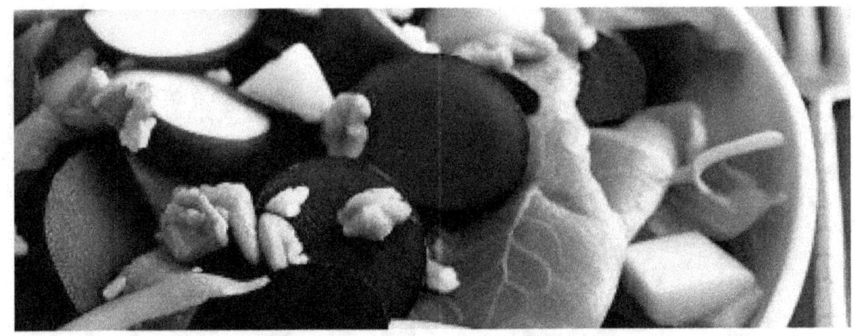

- Roasted beets, sliced
- Mixed salad greens
- Toasted walnuts
- Crumbled Feta cheese
- Apple cider vinegar
- Olive oil
- Dijon mustard
- Honey
- Salt and pepper to taste

Preparation:

1. Place roasted beet slices on a bed of mixed salad leaves.

2. Top with roasted walnuts and feta cheese crumbles.

3. To make the vinaigrette, whisk together apple cider vinegar, olive oil, Dijon mustard, honey, Salt, and pepper in a small basin.

4. Drizzle the vinaigrette over the salad and serve.

Nutritional Values (per Serving):

- 300 calories
- 8g protein
- 6g fiber
- 20g healthy fats
- 25g carbohydrates

Cooking Time: 15 minutes (includes roasting beets and toasting walnuts)

Salad with Spinach and Berries

Ingredients: ★★★★★

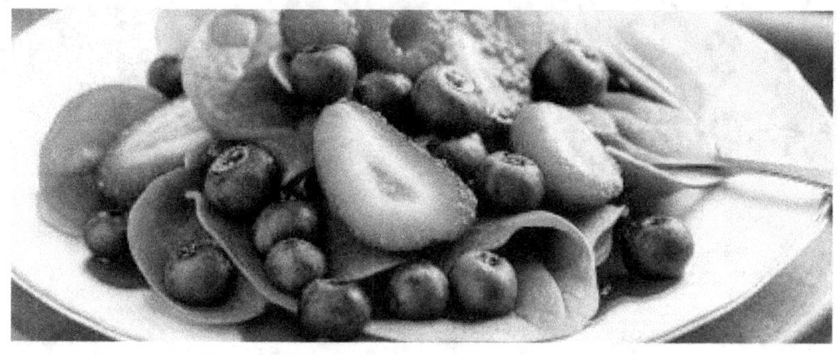

- Fresh spinach leaves
- Mixed berries (strawberries, blueberries, raspberries)
- Finely sliced red Onion
- Feta cheese, crumbled
- Dressing: balsamic vinaigrette
- Optional candied pecans

Preparation:

1. combine fresh spinach leaves, mixed berries, thinly sliced red Onion, and crumbled feta cheese in a mixing dish.

2. Toss gently with the balsamic vinaigrette dressing.

3. If preferred, garnish with candied pecans.

Nutritional Values (per Serving):

- Calories: 200
- Protein: 5g
- Fiber: 4g
- Healthy Fats: 10g
- Carbohydrates: 25g

Time to Cook: 5 minutes (preparation)

Quinoa Tabbouleh Salad

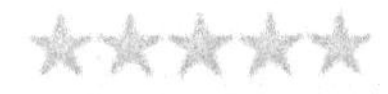

Ingredients:

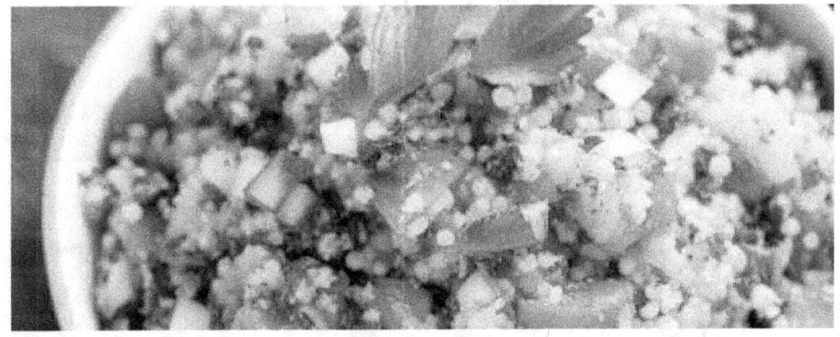

- Quinoa, cooked and chilled
- Cherry tomatoes, halved
- Cucumber, diced
- Fresh parsley, chopped
- Mint leaves, chopped
- Red Onion, finely chopped
- Lemon juice
- Salt & pepper to taste
- Olive oil

Preparation:

1. combine the cooked and cooled quinoa, cherry tomatoes, sliced Cucumber, chopped fresh parsley, mint leaves, and finely chopped red Onion in a mixing dish.
2. Drizzle with olive oil and lemon juice.
3. Season with Salt and pepper to taste.
4. Gently toss the salad until completely incorporated.

Nutritional Values (per Serving):

- Calories: 250
- Protein: 8g
- Fiber: 6g
- Healthy Fats: 10g
- Carbohydrates: 35g

Time to Cook: 15 minutes (quinoa cooking time)

Salad with Mango and Black Beans

Ingredients:

★★★★★

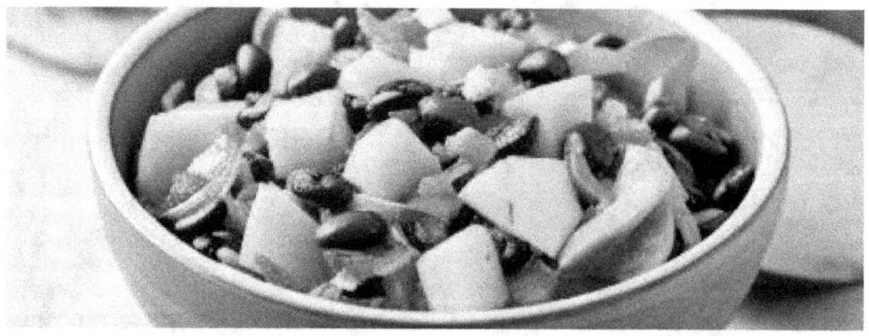

- Tinned, drained, and rinsed black beans
- Mango, diced
- Red bell pepper
- Diced red onion

- Finely chopped fresh cilantro
- Chopped lime juice
- Olive oil, cumin powder
- Salt and pepper to taste

Preparation:

1. combine black beans, diced mango, red bell pepper, finely sliced red Onion, and chopped fresh cilantro in a mixing dish.
2. combine lime juice, olive oil, cumin powder, Salt, and pepper in a small mixing bowl.
3. Pour the dressing over the salad and gently toss to mix.

Nutritional Values (per Serving):

- 220 calories
- 8g protein
- 8g fiber
- 6g healthy fats
- 35g carbohydrates

Time to Cook: 10 minutes (preparation)

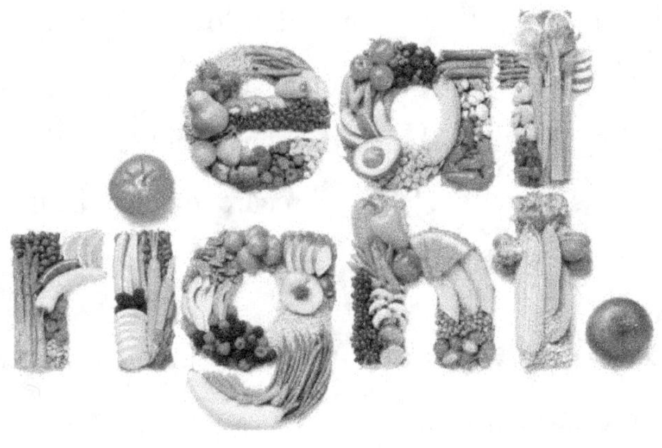

Dear Inspiring Spirits,

Today is the beginning of your incredible path toward bright well-being and boundless vitality. Consider your body to be a blank canvas waiting to be painted with the colors of health and resilience. I'm here to light a fire under you, motivating you to go on an exciting journey of gut health transformation via the power of a great cookbook.

You won't simply find recipes in the vivid pages of this culinary masterpiece; you'll also discover the alchemy of self-love and longevity. This cookbook is more than just a compilation of recipes; it's your ticket to a symphony of flavors that dance in unison with your stomach. Every meal is a declaration—a vow to nourish your body's unique ecology.

Take this journey with enthusiasm! Allow each recipe to be a watershed moment, each mouthful a tribute to your commitment to a dazzling, unstoppable self. You're not simply cooking; you're creating a resilient legacy. Prepare to celebrate the victory of a healthier, more energized life!

Joan Your Motivational Guide to Gut Greatness, with endless encouragement

Chapter 8:

Meat And Poultry

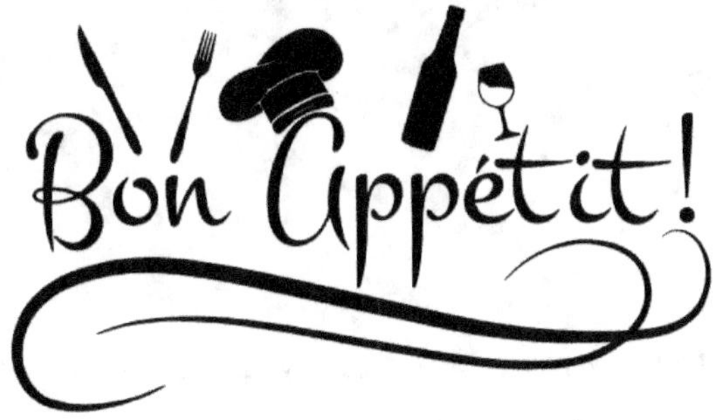

Savory Indulgence: Meat and Poultry, a chapter meant to satisfy carnivorous urges and enrich your dining experience, ushering you into gastronomic indulgence. This chapter honors the rich, substantial tastes that meat and poultry bring, with each recipe demonstrating the technique of creating delicious, tasty meals.

"Savory Indulgence: Meat and Poultry" invites you to cherish every moment and enjoy indulging in the savory side of life.

Probiotic Marinade for Grilled Chicken

Ingredients: ★★★★★

- Chicken breasts
- Yogurt (probiotic-rich)

- Garlic, minced
- Lemon juice
- Fresh thyme, chopped
- Olive oil,
- Salt and pepper to taste

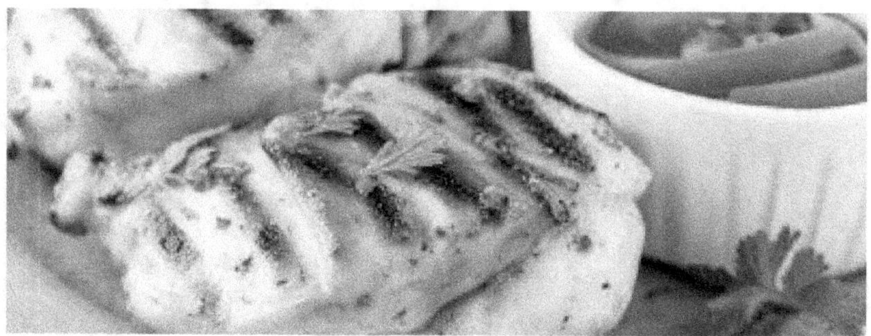

Preparation:

1. To make the marinade, combine yogurt, minced Garlic, lemon juice, chopped fresh thyme, olive oil, Salt, and pepper in a mixing dish.
2. Coat the chicken breasts evenly with the marinade.
3. Marinate for at least 2 hours or overnight in the refrigerator.
4. Preheat the grill and cook the chicken until thoroughly done and the exterior has a beautiful char.

Nutritional Values (per Serving):

- Calories: 300
- Protein: 35g
-
- Probiotics for gut health
- Healthy Fats: 10g

Time to cook: 15-20 minutes (including marination)

Stuffed Pepper with Turkey and Quinoa

Ingredients:

★★★★★

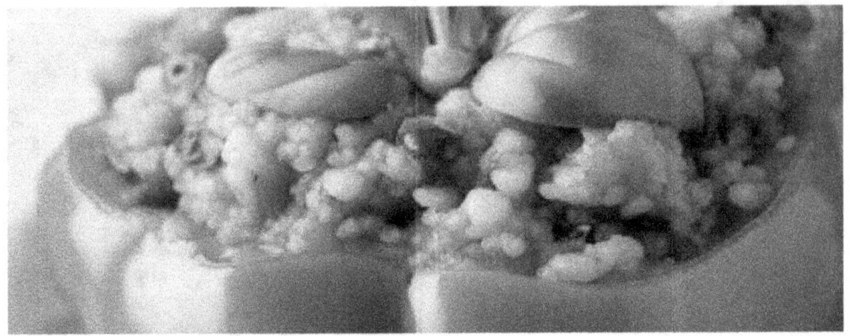

- Halved bell peppers with seeds removed
- Ground turkey
- Quinoa, cooked
- Onion, finely chopped
- Garlic, minced
- Tomato sauce
- Seasonings from Italy
- Shredded mozzarella cheese (optional, for topping)
- Salt & pepper to taste

Preparation:

1. Preheat the oven to 375 degrees Fahrenheit (190 degrees Celsius).
2. Sauté finely chopped Onion and minced Garlic in a skillet until softened.
3. Cook until the ground turkey is browned.
4. Combine cooked quinoa, tomato sauce, Italian seasoning, Salt, and pepper in a mixing bowl.
5. Spoon the mixture into the halves of the bell peppers.

6. Garnish with shredded mozzarella cheese if desired.

7. Bake for 25-30 minutes until the peppers are soft.

Nutritional Values (per Serving):

- 300 calories
- 25g protein
- 5g fiber
- 8g healthy fats
- 30g carbohydrates

30 minutes total cooking time (including baking time)

Stir-fry Lean Beef and Vegetables

Ingredients: ★★★★★

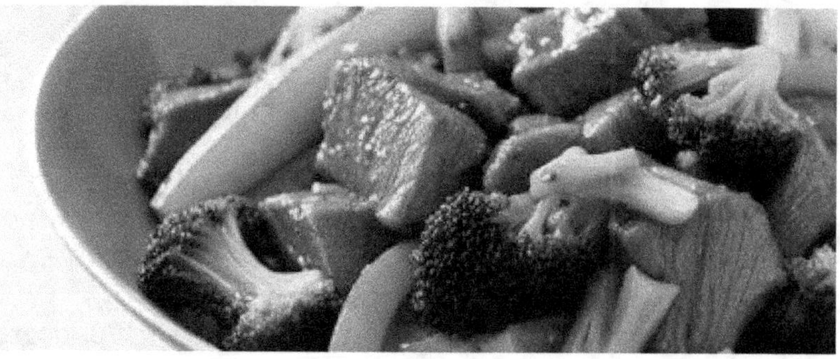

- Lean beef strips, mixed veggies (broccoli, bell peppers, carrots), and soy sauce
- Garlic, chopped
- Ginger, grated
- Sesame oil, olive oil
- Salt and pepper to taste

Preparation:

1. Heat olive oil in a wok or pan and sauté minced garlic and grated ginger until aromatic.
2. Stir-fry the lean beef strips until they are browned.
3. Continue to stir-fry the mixed veggies until crisp-tender.
4. Toss in the soy sauce and sesame oil to cover evenly.
5. Season with Salt and pepper to taste.

Nutritional Values (per Serving):

- 350 Calories
- 30g Protein
- 6g Fiber
- 10g Healthy Fats
- 25g Carbohydrates

Time to cook: 15 minutes

One Pot Garlic Chicken 

Ingredients:

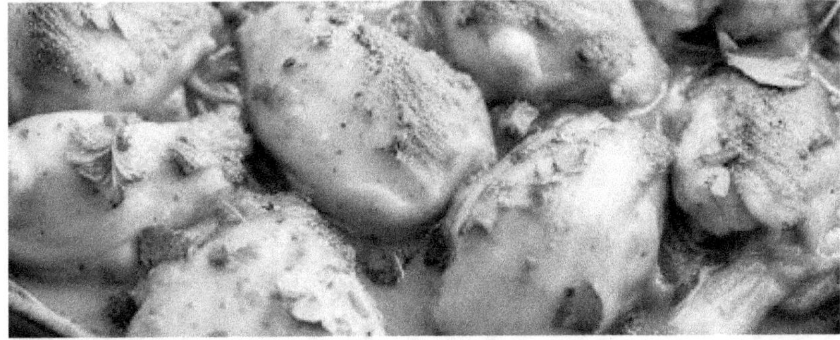

- Chicken thighs, bone-in
- Skin-on baby potatoes
- Split carrots
- Sliced Garlic
- Entire cloves
- Olive oil

- Fresh thyme
- Chicken broth
- Salt and pepper to taste

Preparation:

1. Heat the olive oil in a big saucepan and brown the chicken thighs on both sides.
2. Stir in the young potatoes, carrots, garlic cloves, and fresh thyme.
3. Add the chicken broth and season with Salt and pepper to taste.
4. Cover and simmer for 30-40 minutes until the chicken is cooked and the potatoes are soft.

Nutritional Values (per Serving):

- Calories: 400
- Protein: 30g
- Fiber: 6g
- Healthy Fats: 12g
- Carbohydrates: 30g

Time to cook: 40 minutes

Skewers of Tandoori Chicken 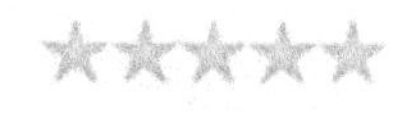

Ingredients:

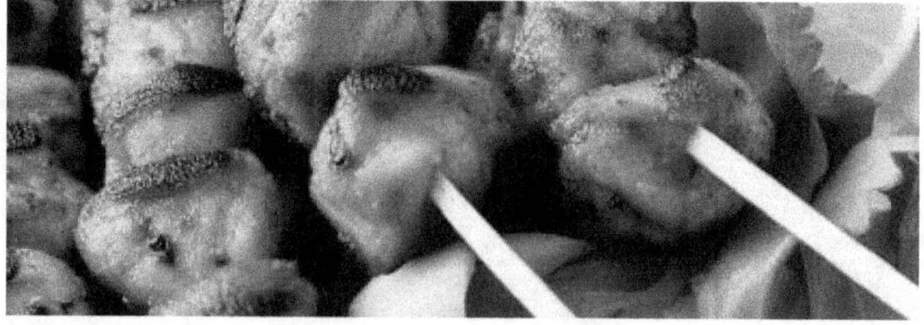

- Chicken breast, sliced into cubes
- Yogurt, and a tandoori spice combination.
- Garlic, chopped
- Ginger, grated
- Lemon juice
- Olive oil
- Salt, and pepper to taste

Preparation:

1. To make the marinade, combine yogurt, tandoori spice mix, minced Garlic, grated ginger, lemon juice, olive oil, Salt, and pepper in a mixing bowl.
2. Marinate the chicken cubes in the marinade for at least 2 hours or overnight.
3. Skewer marinated chicken on skewers.
4. Grill the skewers until the chicken is cooked and the exterior has a beautiful sear.

Nutritional Values (per Serving):

- Calories: 250
- Protein: 30g
- Healthy Fats: 10g
- Carbohydrates: 5g

Time to cook: 15 minutes (grilling time)

Lemon Herb Grilled Chicken Breast

Ingredients: ★★★★★

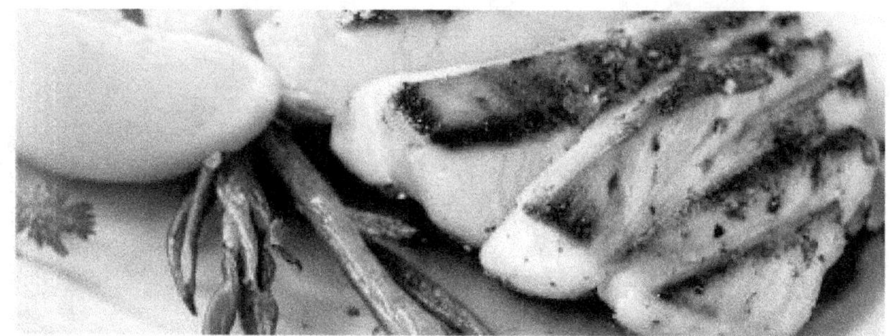

- 4 skinless, boneless chicken breasts
- 2 (juiced) lemons
- 3 tablespoons olive oil
- 2 minced garlic cloves
- 1 teaspoon dried oregano
- 1 teaspoon dried thyme
- Season with salt and black pepper to taste.
- Garnish with fresh parsley (optional)

Preparation:

1. Combine lemon juice, olive oil, minced garlic, dried oregano, dried thyme, salt, and pepper in a mixing bowl.
2. Marinate the chicken in half of the marinade for at least 30 minutes, preferably overnight for a more flavorful result.
3. Preheat the grill to medium-high.
4. Grill the chicken for 6-8 minutes each side, or until it reaches an internal temperature of 165°F (74°C).
5. During the last five minutes of cooking, baste with the remaining marinade.
6. Allow the chicken to rest before serving. If desired, garnish with fresh parsley.

Per serving nutritional value:

- Calorie count: 250 kcal
- 30g protein
- Fat: ~12g
- 5g carbohydrate
- 1g dietary fiber

Time to Cook: 30 minutes to overnight marinating

12-16 minutes grilling

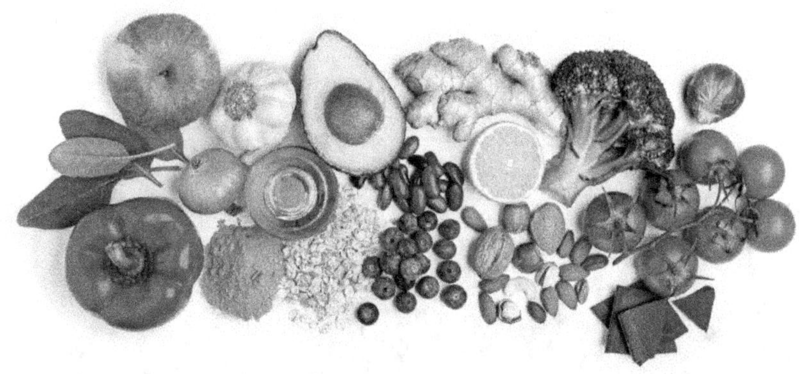

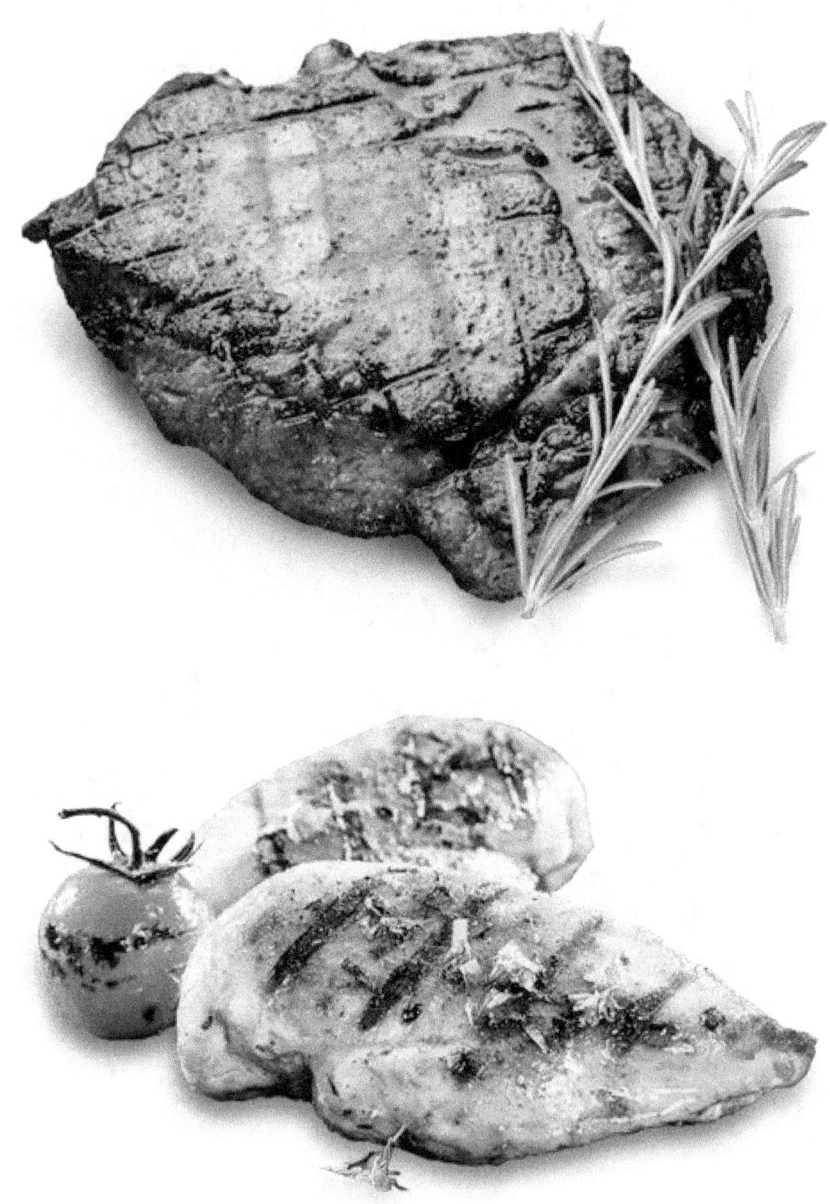

Chapter 9

Seafood

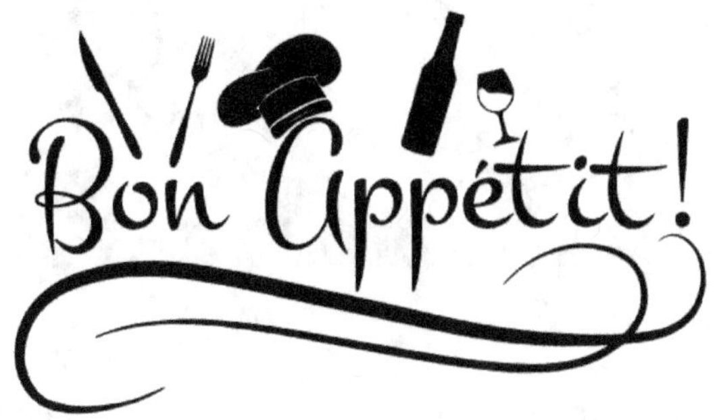

Dive into the culinary depths with "Ocean's Bounty: Seafood," a symphony of tastes featuring the wonders of the sea. This chapter delves into the varied and wonderful world of seafood with recipes highlighting ocean treats' freshness, variety, and nutritional richness.

Prepare for a gastronomic journey where every taste celebrates the sea's riches.

Seared Tuna with Ginger and Soy

Ingredients:

★★★★★

- Ahi tuna steaks Soy sauce

- Fresh ginger, grated

- Garlic, minced
- Sesame oil
- Green onions sliced

- Sesame seeds (for decoration)
- Lime wedges (for serving)

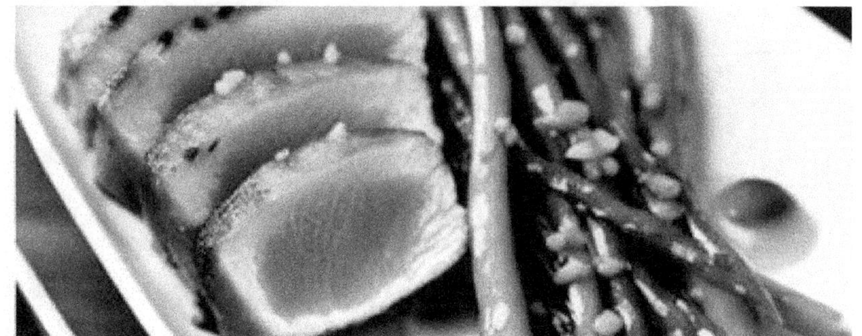

Preparation:

1. To make the marinade, combine soy sauce, grated fresh ginger, minced Garlic, and sesame oil in a mixing bowl.
2. Coat the tuna steaks in the marinade and let aside for 15-30 minutes.
3. Preheat a skillet or grill to high heat.
4. Sea the tuna for 1-2 minutes on each side for a rare to medium-rare outcome.
5. Serve with chopped green onions and sesame seeds as garnish.
6. Garnish with lime wedges.

Nutritional Values (per Serving):

- Calories: 200
- Protein: 25g

- Healthy Fats: 8g
- Carbohydrates: 2g

Time to cook: 5 minutes

Garlic and Lemon Shrimp Skewers

Ingredients:

★★★★★

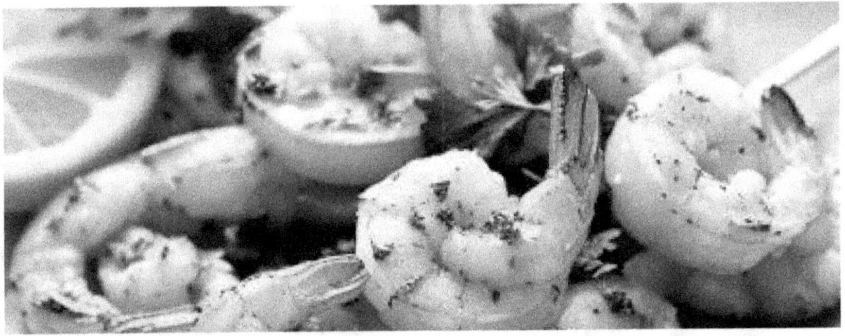

- Peeled and deveined shrimp
- Minced Garlic
- Lemon zest
- Lemon juice
- Olive oil
- Chopped fresh parsley
- Salt and pepper to taste.

Preparation:

1. To make the marinade, add minced Garlic, lemon zest, lemon juice, olive oil, chopped fresh parsley, Salt, and pepper in a mixing dish.
2. Thread the shrimp onto skewers and brush with the marinade. Allow them to marinade for 15 to 30 minutes.
3. Grill the shrimp skewers on each side for 2-3 minutes or until they are opaque.
4. Serve right away.

Nutritional Values (per Serving):

- 150 Calories
- 20g Protein
- 8g Healthy Fats
- 2g Carbohydrates

Time to cook: 6 minutes (grilling time)

Cod Baked with Herbs and Lemon

Ingredients:

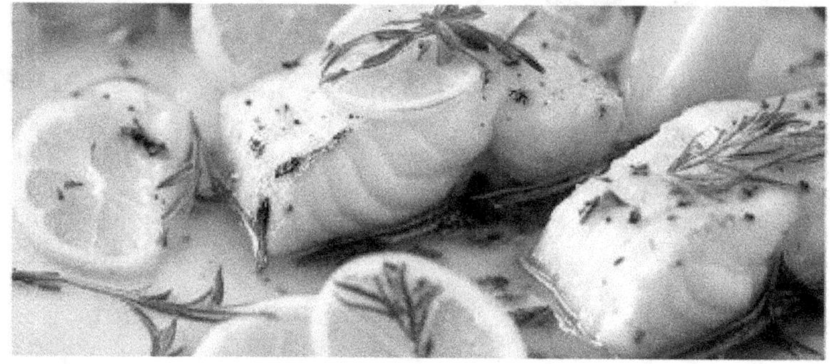

- Cod fillets
- Fresh herbs (such as parsley, dill, and thyme) sliced
- Garlic, minced
- Lemon zest
- Lemon juice.
- Extra virgin olive oil
- Salt and pepper to taste

Preparation:

1. Preheat the oven to 375 degrees Fahrenheit (190 degrees Celsius).

2. Arrange the fish fillets on a baking sheet.

3. To make the herb marinade, combine chopped fresh herbs, minced Garlic, lemon zest, lemon juice, olive oil, Salt, and pepper in a mixing dish.

4. Brush the herb marinade over the fish fillets.

5. Bake for 15-20 minutes or until the fish is flaky and well-cooked.

Nutritional Values (per Serving):

- Calories: 180
- Protein: 25g
- Healthy Fats: 8g
- Carbohydrates: 1g

Time to cook: 20 minutes

Tilapia Coconut-Curry ★★★★★

Ingredients:

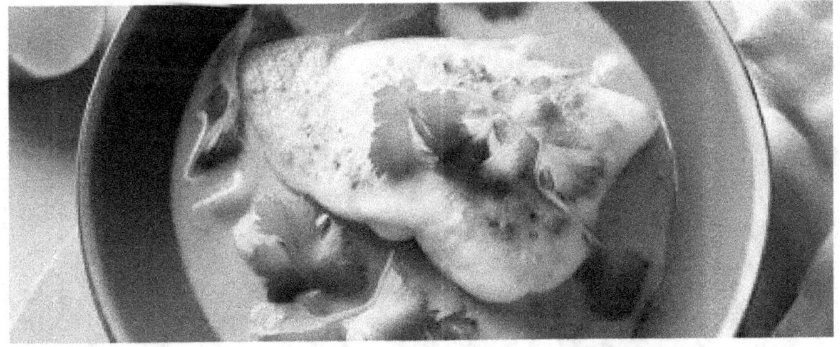

- Tilapia fillets
- Coconut milk
- Red curry paste
- Garlic, minced
- Ginger, grated
- Lime juice
- Fresh cilantro, chopped
- Salt and pepper to taste

Preparation:

1. To make the marinade, combine coconut milk, red curry paste, minced Garlic, grated ginger, lime juice, chopped fresh cilantro, Salt, and pepper in a mixing bowl.

2. Marinate the tilapia fillets in the curry marinade for 15-30 minutes.

3. Preheat the oven to 375 degrees Fahrenheit (190 degrees Celsius).

4. Bake for 15-20 minutes or until the tilapia flakes easily with a fork.

Nutritional Values (per Serving):

- Calories: 220
- Protein: 20g
- Healthy Fats: 15g
- Carbohydrates: 5g

Time to cook: 20 minutes

Lemon Herb Grilled Swordfish ★★★★★

Ingredients:

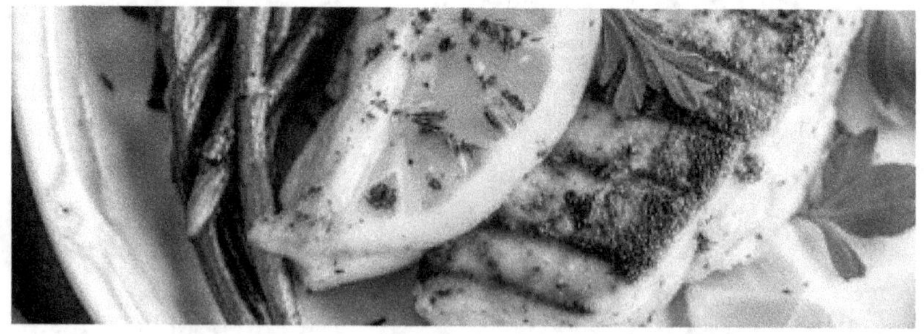

- Swordfish steaks
- Lemon, thinly sliced
- Fresh herbs (rosemary, thyme, and oregano), chopped
- Garlic, minced
- Extra virgin olive oil
- Salt and pepper to taste

Preparation:

1. Heat the grill to medium-high.
2. To make the herb marinade, combine chopped fresh herbs, minced Garlic, olive oil, Salt, and pepper in a mixing dish.
3. Marinate the swordfish steaks in the herb marinade.
4. Place a slice of lemon on top of each swordfish steak.
5. Grill the swordfish for 3-4 minutes per side or until cooked through and charred.

Nutritional Values (per Serving):

- Calories: 250
- Protein: 30g
- Healthy Fats: 12g
- Carbohydrates: 2g

Time to cook: 8-10 minutes

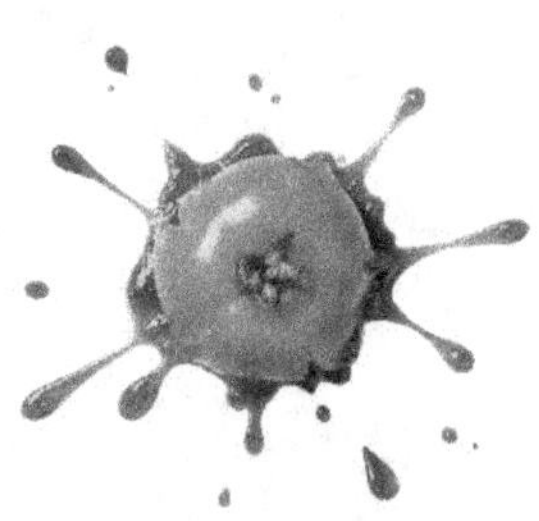

Dear Respected Readers,

Starting a journey to improve your gut health is a strong step toward self-love and energy. Consider a life in which every meal is an opportunity to nurture not just your body, but also your spirit. I am honored to accompany you on this transforming journey, where the pages of a cookbook serve as your road map to gut health paradise.

Discover the magic of whole foods in each dish to revitalize and stimulate your digestive system. Every component is proof that a symphony of tastes may heal from inside. As you begin on this culinary adventure, keep in mind that you are making a masterpiece for your own well-being.

You're not simply cooking with resolve and the correct ingredients; you're manifesting a dazzling, energetic version of yourself. Take advantage of this chance to learn the skill of mindful eating and watch the tremendous transformation that takes place inside you.

To a life of vigorous health and gastronomic delight,

Joan.

Appendix:

Handy Resources

Shopping List for Pantry Staples

Pantry Staples for a Gut-Healthy Kitchen:

1. **Grains:**

- Quinoa
- Brown rice
- Oats (rolled or steel-cut)
- Whole-grain pasta

2. **Legumes:**

- Lentils (red and green)
- Chickpeas
- Black beans

3. **Healthy Fats:**

- Olive oil (extra virgin)
- Avocado oil
- Nuts (almonds, walnuts)
- Seeds (chia seeds, flaxseeds)

4. **Herbs and Spices:**

- Fresh herbs (parsley, cilantro, thyme, rosemary)
- Ground turmeric
- Cumin
- Paprika
- Garlic powder
- Ginger (fresh or ground)

5. **Proteins:**

- Lean poultry (chicken, turkey)
- Lean meats (beef, pork)
- Fish fillets (salmon, cod, tilapia)
- Eggs

6. **Dairy and Dairy Alternatives:**

- Greek yogurt (unsweetened)
- Almond milk or other plant-based milk

7. **Fresh Produce:**

- Leafy greens (spinach, kale)
- Berries (blueberries, strawberries)
- Citrus fruits (lemons, limes)
- Avocados
- Bell peppers
- Tomatoes

8. **Canned Goods:**

- Canned tomatoes
- Coconut milk
- Black beans (canned, no added salt)
- Chickpeas (canned, no added salt)
- Tuna (canned in water)

9. **Whole Grains:**

- Whole-grain bread
- Whole-grain tortillas

10. **Condiments:**

- Soy sauce (low sodium)

- Olive oil-based vinaigrette
- Mustard (Dijon or whole grain)
- Red curry paste
- Honey

11. **Extras:**

- Dark chocolate (70% cocoa or higher)
- Green tea

Ingredient Substitutions and Alternatives

Alternatives to Flour:

To increase fiber and nutrients, replace refined flour with whole grain flour such as almond, coconut, or oat flour.

Sugar substitutes:

Substitute natural sweeteners such as honey, maple syrup, or agave nectar for refined sugar to encourage a healthy gut.

Dairy Alternatives:

For people who are lactose intolerant, choose lactose-free or plant-based alternatives such as almond milk, coconut milk, or soy milk.

Oils for cooking:

For anti-inflammatory characteristics, replace vegetable oils with gut-friendly choices such as olive, avocado, or coconut oil.

Sources of protein:

To minimize saturated fats and boost intestinal health, replace red meat with lean chicken, fish, or plant-based proteins like tofu, tempeh, or lentils.

Gluten-Free Alternatives:

For people who are gluten intolerant, try gluten-free grains such as quinoa, brown rice, or buckwheat.

Low-FODMAP Options:

Consider green beans, zucchini, or bell peppers instead of high-FODMAP veggies for those following a low-FODMAP diet.

Foods High in Probiotics:

To improve the gut microbiota, replace fermented foods like sauerkraut, kimchi, or kefir with standard sides.

Alternatives for seeds and nuts:

If allergies are an issue, substitute sunflower or chia seeds with nuts like almond butter or sunflower seed butter.

Dairy with Low Lactose Content:

For people who are lactose intolerant, choose lactose-free or low-lactose dairy products such as lactose-free yogurt or hard cheeses.

Artificial Ingredients:

Reduce artificial recipe ingredients by integrating natural tastes like herbs, spices, and citrus fruits.

Snacks Made from Whole Foods:

To improve intestinal health, replace processed snacks with nutritious foods such as fresh fruits, vegetables, and nuts.

Individual tolerances vary, so listen to your body and make modifications depending on your unique requirements and preferences. For individualized guidance, always visit a healthcare practitioner or a nutritionist.

Cooking Techniques for Sensitive Stomachs

Steaming:

Steaming is accessible on the stomach and maintains nutrients without adding fat. For a stomach-friendly dinner, steamed veggies, seafood, or grains like rice.

Poaching:

Poaching involves boiling food in liquid to keep it delicate. To aid digestion, poach chicken, fish, or eggs in broth.

Slow cooker:

Slow cooking at low temperatures helps flavors mingle and break down fibers in difficult materials, simplifying digestion.

Pureeing and blending:

Make smooth soups, purees, or smoothies to help folks with sensitive stomachs digest. This method is ideal for integrating fruits and vegetables.

Broiling or grilling:

Cooking over direct heat quickly locks in flavors without additional oil. For a lighter alternative, use lean proteins such as chicken or fish.

Baking:

Baking at lower temperatures with little additional fat can be a gentle cooking technique. Choose roasted veggies, lean meats, or fruit desserts instead.

Sautéing with Little Oil:

Sautéing lightly with a tiny amount of oil helps to maintain taste without overpowering the stomach. Make use of heart-healthy oils such as olive or avocado oil.

Marinating:

Marinating meats in acidic solutions (such as citrus or vinegar) before cooking can help break down proteins and make them more digestible.

Meals that are small and frequent:

Smaller, more frequent meals throughout the day are preferable to larger, more frequent meals. This method allows for better portion control and digestion.

Avoiding Hot Foods:

Those with sensitive stomachs may benefit from decreasing or avoiding spicy meals. To flavor meals, use milder herbs and spices.

Skin and Seed Removal:

Removing rough skins and seeds from fruits and vegetables can simplify digestion.

Including Ginger and Mint:

Ginger and mint both have digestive properties. To ease the stomach, use them in dishes or make drinks.

Cooking strategies for sensitive stomachs must focus on approaches that enhance tastes and textures without discomfort. Experimenting with these moderate ways can help to make cooking more fun and palatable.

Meal Planning with Digestive Conditions

Probiotics should be included:

Consume probiotic-rich foods such as yogurt, kefir, or fermented vegetables to encourage a healthy gut flora balance.

Foods High in Fiber:

Eat high-fiber meals such as whole grains, fruits, and vegetables to encourage regular bowel movements and general gut health.

Proteins that are low in fat:

To get vital amino acids without adding fat, use lean protein sources like poultry, fish, tofu, or lentils.

Low-FODMAP Alternatives:

If you have IBS, you should consider a low-FODMAP diet. Include low-FODMAP fruits (such as berries), vegetables (such as spinach), and grains (such as quinoa).

Hydration:

Drink plenty of water to aid digestion. Water, herbal teas, fruit, and herb-infused water are all wonderful options.

Meals that are small and frequent:

To minimize intestinal overload, plan smaller, more frequent meals. This can aid with symptom management and digestion.

Limit your intake of processed foods:

Reduce your intake of processed and high-fat meals, which might be difficult to digest. For improved gut health, choose whole, unprocessed foods.

Gentle Cooking Methods:

To improve digestibility, use moderate cooking methods such as steaming, poaching, or slow cooking.

Journaling about Food:

Maintain a food journal to keep track of your meals and identify trigger foods. This can assist you in understanding your body's reactions and making educated decisions.

Eating with Intention:

Practice attentive eating by properly chewing your meal and appreciating each bite. This promotes digestion and keeps you from overeating.

Digestive Aids should be included:

Include natural digestive aides in your meals or drinks, such as ginger, peppermint, or fennel.

The plate is balanced:

Prepare balanced meals that include protein, healthy fats, and complex carbs to give continuous energy and promote digestion.

Caffeine and alcohol should be avoided:

Caffeine and alcohol are both diuretics that can irritate the digestive tract. Alternative drinks include herbal teas and water.

Consult with an Expert:

To build a tailored meal plan, consult a healthcare provider or registered dietitian specializing in digestive health.

A judicious blend of nutritional meals, mindful eating habits, and consideration of individual sensitivities is required when tailoring your meal plan to suit digestive issues. Reassess and change your strategy regularly based on your body's responses, and communicate with healthcare specialists for continuous assistance.

7 Days Meal Planning Sample

Day 1:

Breakfast - Berry-Probiotic Smoothie Bowl

Lunch - Protein-Packed Lentil and Vegetable Wrap

Dinner - Baked Salmon with Lemon and Dill

Day 2:

Breakfast - Overnight Oats with Gut-Friendly Seeds

Lunch - Quinoa Salad with Fermented Veggies

Dinner - Vegetarian Stir-Fry with Tofu

Day 3:

Breakfast - Spinach and Feta Breakfast Muffins

Lunch - Chicken and Avocado Quinoa Bowl

Dinner - Baked Cod with Herbs and Lemon

Day 4:

Breakfast - Chia Seed Pudding Parfait

Lunch - Mediterranean Chickpea Salad

Dinner - Turmeric-Ginger Chicken Skewers

Day 5:

Breakfast - Quinoa Breakfast Bowl

Lunch - Sweet Potato and Kale Salad

Dinner - Quinoa and Black Bean Stuffed Peppers

Day 6:

Breakfast - Lemon Herb Grilled Swordfish

Lunch - Roasted Chickpeas with Spices

Dinner - Brown Rice Pilaf with Mixed Vegetables

Day 7:

Breakfast - Tandoori Chicken Skewers

Lunch - Mashed Cauliflower with Turmeric

Dinner - Salmon and Asparagus Foil Packets

Remember to adjust portion sizes based on individual needs and consult with a healthcare professional or nutritionist for personalized advice. Enjoy your delicious and gut-healthy meals!

Glossary of Terms and Ingredients

Probiotics:

Beneficial bacteria that are alive and create a healthy balance of microorganisms in the gut. Fermented foods such as yogurt, kefir, and sauerkraut contain probiotics.

Prebiotics:

Nondigestible fibers that nourish and encourage probiotic development in the gut. Foods containing it include garlic, onions, and bananas.

Microbiome:

The vast collection of microorganisms lives in the digestive system, including bacteria, viruses, fungi, and others.

Fiber:

Plant material that is indigestible and improves bowel regularity and intestinal health. Found in fruits and vegetables, as well as entire grains.

Fermentation:

The breakdown of carbohydrates by bacteria into acids or gases. Fermented foods such as kimchi and kombucha are commonly fermented.

Enzymes Digestive:

Proteins that help macronutrients (proteins, fats, and carbs) break down into smaller, more absorbable components.

Fatty Acids Omega-3:

Anti-inflammatory essential fatty acids are found in fatty fish (salmon, mackerel), flaxseeds, and walnuts.

Polyphenols:

Plant-based antioxidant chemicals, such as berries, green tea, and dark chocolate, promote intestinal health.

Lactobacillus:

A genus of bacteria found in yogurt and other fermented foods is recognized for fostering a healthy gut environment.

Bifidobacterium:

Another beneficial type of bacteria is found in fermented dairy products and certain supplements.

Glutamine:

An amino acid is vital for gut health because it helps keep the intestinal lining intact.

Leaky Gut Syndrome (LGS):

A disorder in which the intestinal lining becomes more porous, potentially admitting toxic chemicals into the circulation.

Inulin:

A prebiotic fiber found in foods such as chicory root, garlic, and onions that promotes the growth of good gut flora.

Turmeric:

Curcumin, the main ingredient in turmeric, is anti-inflammatory and may aid gut health.

Ginger:

A root used in drinks and cooking for its anti-inflammatory and digestive qualities.

Broth de boeuf:

A broth created by boiling animal bones and connective tissue that is high in nutrients such as collagen and gelatin and may help with digestive health.

Miso:

A Japanese condiment made by fermenting soybeans is frequently used to make a delicious soup containing probiotics.

Vinegar of Apple Cider:

Fermented apple juice may aid digestion and intestinal health when drunk in moderation.

Understanding these words and including associated foods in your diet can help you live a more gut-healthy lifestyle. Always seek tailored guidance from a healthcare professional.

For further Questions and advice reach out on
joanmilonehelpdesk@gmail.com

Thank You

I'm writing this with a heart full of gratitude for your kind words and the time you took to read my book, knowing that my words have resonated with you is a reward beyond measure. Thank you again for your appreciation and for being a part of this literary journey.

Warmly,

Joan

HAPPY COOKING!!

>>> 30 Days
Meal Planner

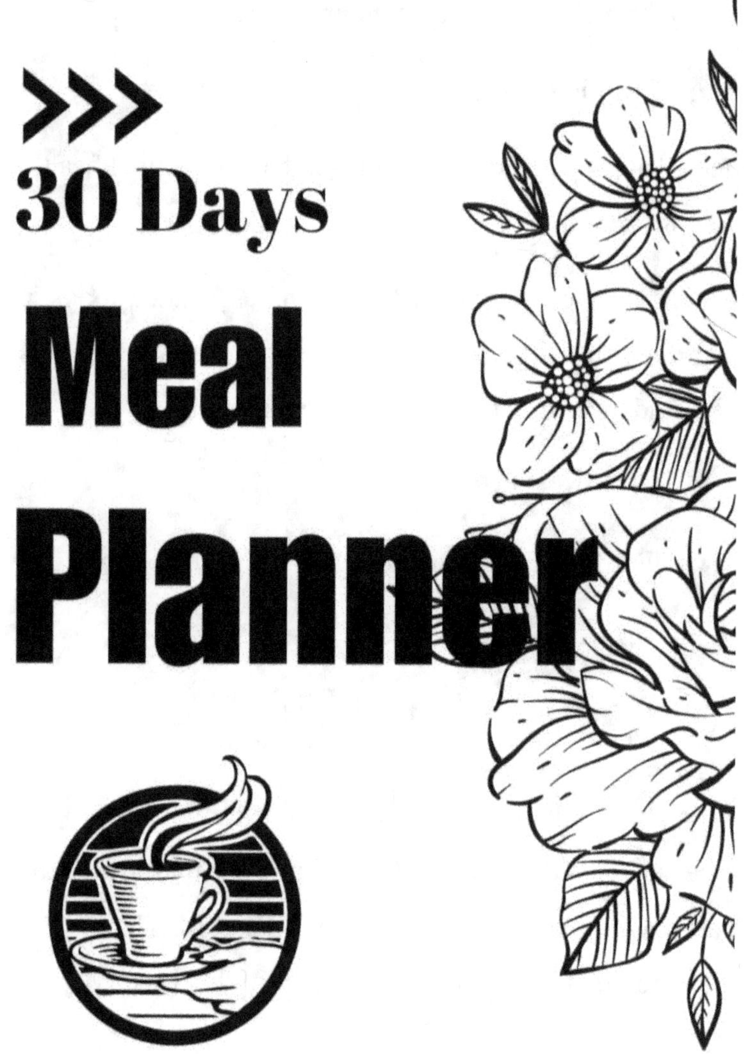

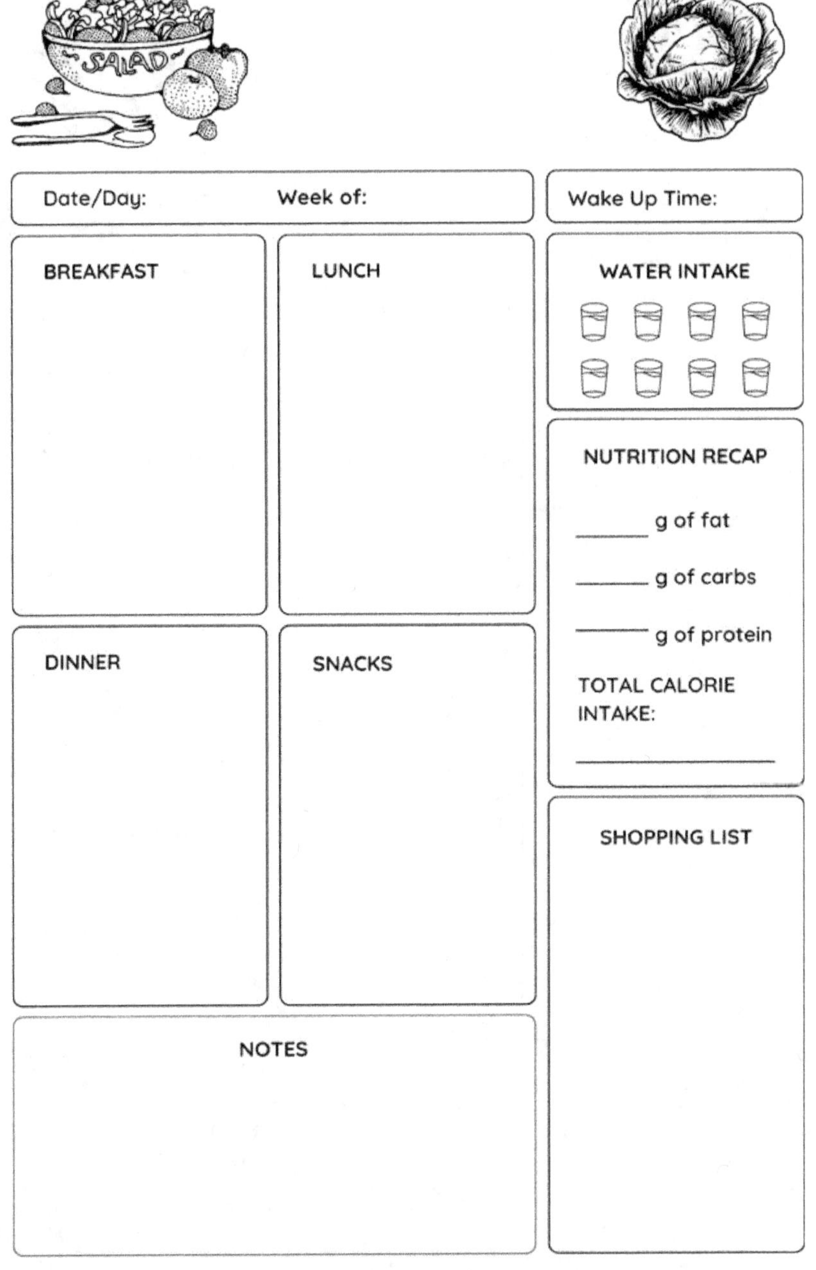

Date/Day: Week of:

Wake Up Time:

BREAKFAST

LUNCH

WATER INTAKE

NUTRITION RECAP

________ g of fat

________ g of carbs

________ g of protein

TOTAL CALORIE INTAKE:

____

DINNER

SNACKS

SHOPPING LIST

NOTES

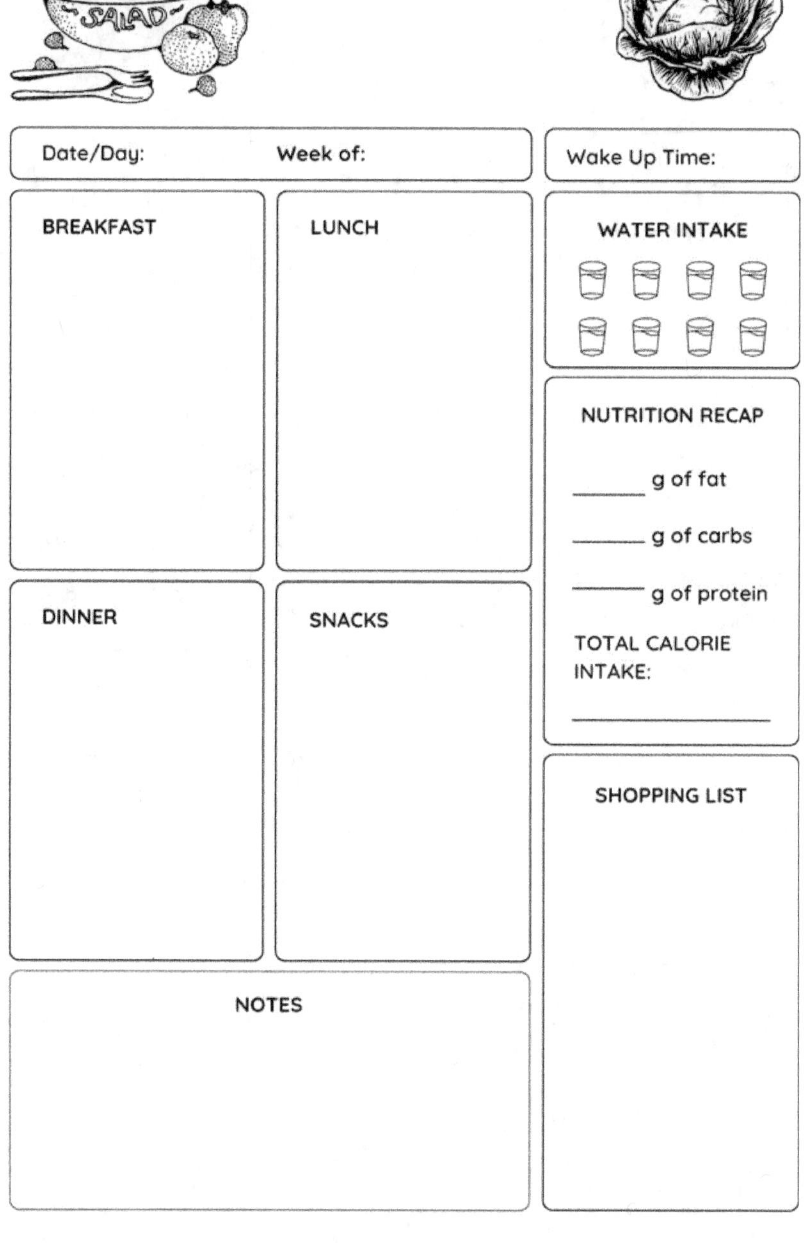

Date/Day: Week of:

Wake Up Time:

BREAKFAST

LUNCH

WATER INTAKE

NUTRITION RECAP

_______ g of fat

_______ g of carbs

_______ g of protein

TOTAL CALORIE INTAKE:

____

DINNER

SNACKS

SHOPPING LIST

NOTES

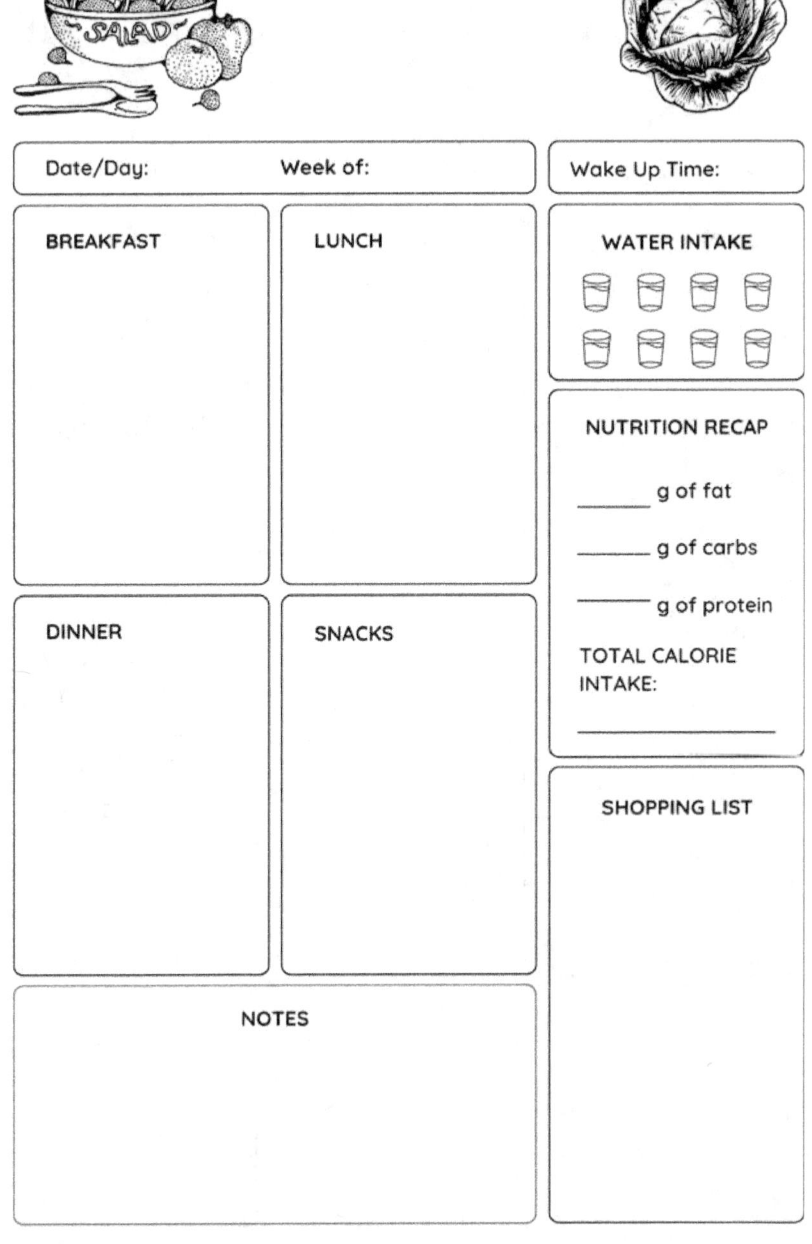

Date/Day: Week of:

Wake Up Time:

BREAKFAST

LUNCH

WATER INTAKE

NUTRITION RECAP

________ g of fat

________ g of carbs

________ g of protein

TOTAL CALORIE INTAKE:

DINNER

SNACKS

SHOPPING LIST

NOTES

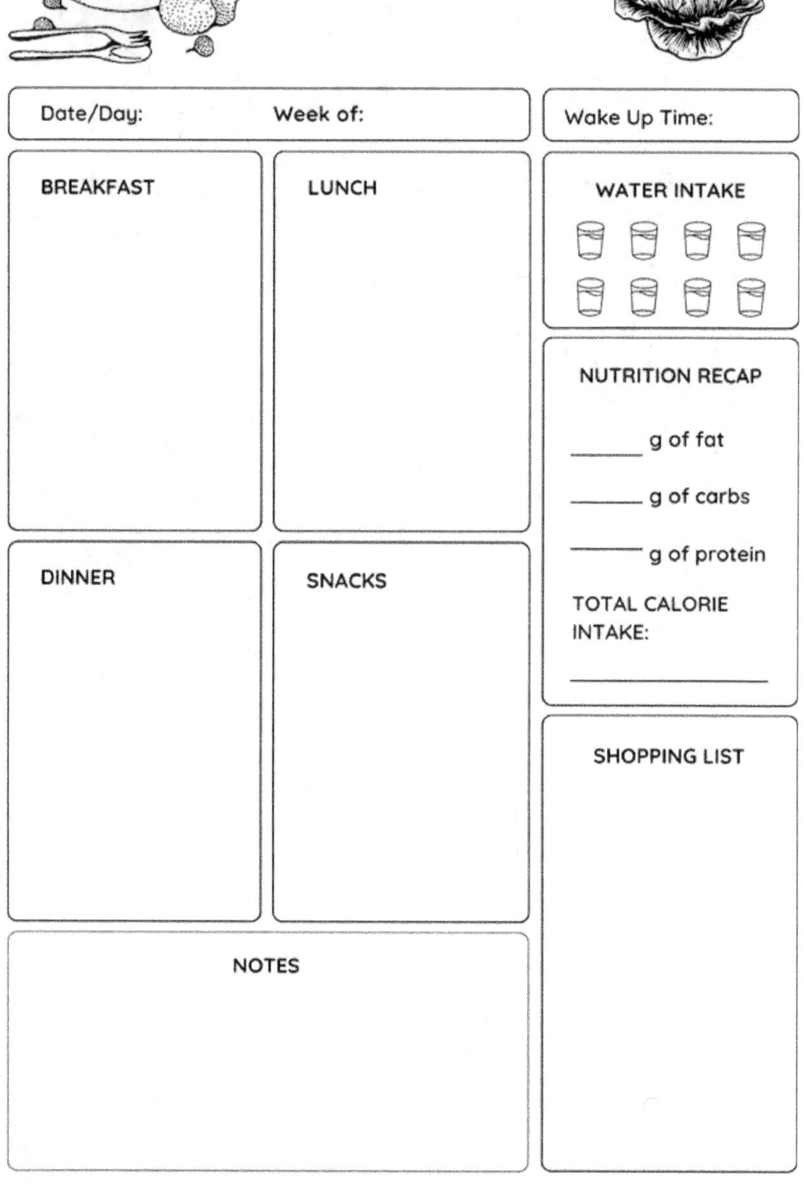

| Date/Day: | Week of: | Wake Up Time: |

BREAKFAST

LUNCH

WATER INTAKE

NUTRITION RECAP

_______ g of fat

_______ g of carbs

_______ g of protein

TOTAL CALORIE INTAKE:

____

DINNER

SNACKS

SHOPPING LIST

NOTES

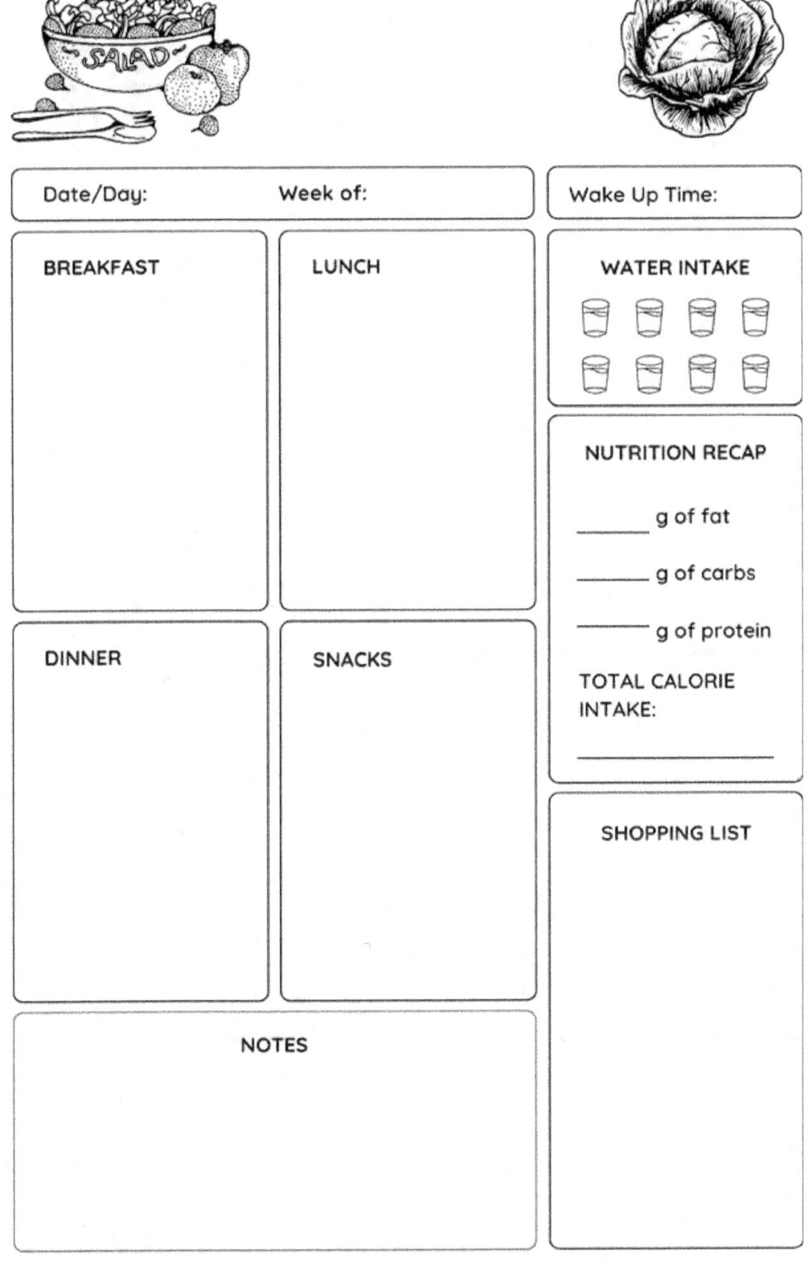

Date/Day: Week of:

Wake Up Time:

BREAKFAST

LUNCH

WATER INTAKE

NUTRITION RECAP

______ g of fat

______ g of carbs

______ g of protein

TOTAL CALORIE INTAKE:

____

DINNER

SNACKS

SHOPPING LIST

NOTES

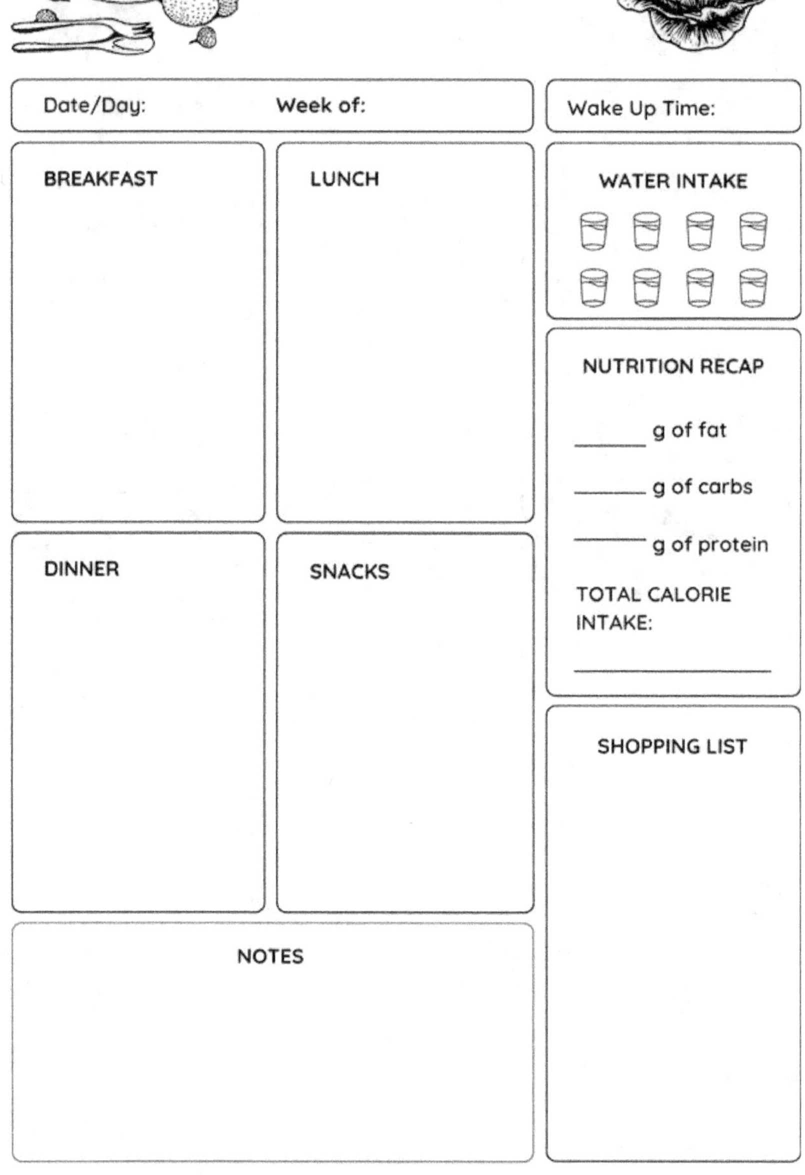

| Date/Day: | Week of: | Wake Up Time: |

BREAKFAST

LUNCH

WATER INTAKE

NUTRITION RECAP

_______ g of fat

_______ g of carbs

_______ g of protein

TOTAL CALORIE INTAKE:

____

DINNER

SNACKS

SHOPPING LIST

NOTES

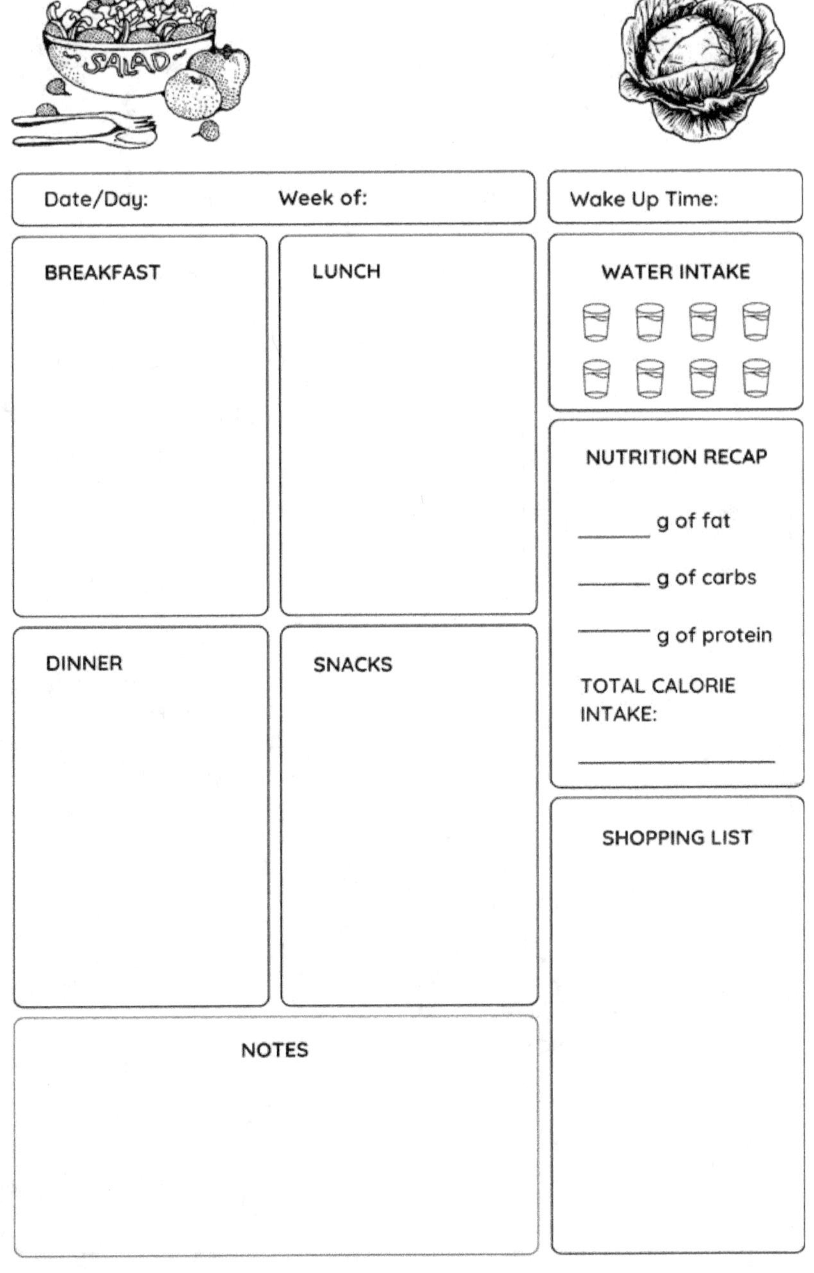

| Date/Day: | Week of: | Wake Up Time: |

BREAKFAST

LUNCH

WATER INTAKE

NUTRITION RECAP

_______ g of fat

_______ g of carbs

_______ g of protein

TOTAL CALORIE INTAKE:

____

DINNER

SNACKS

SHOPPING LIST

NOTES

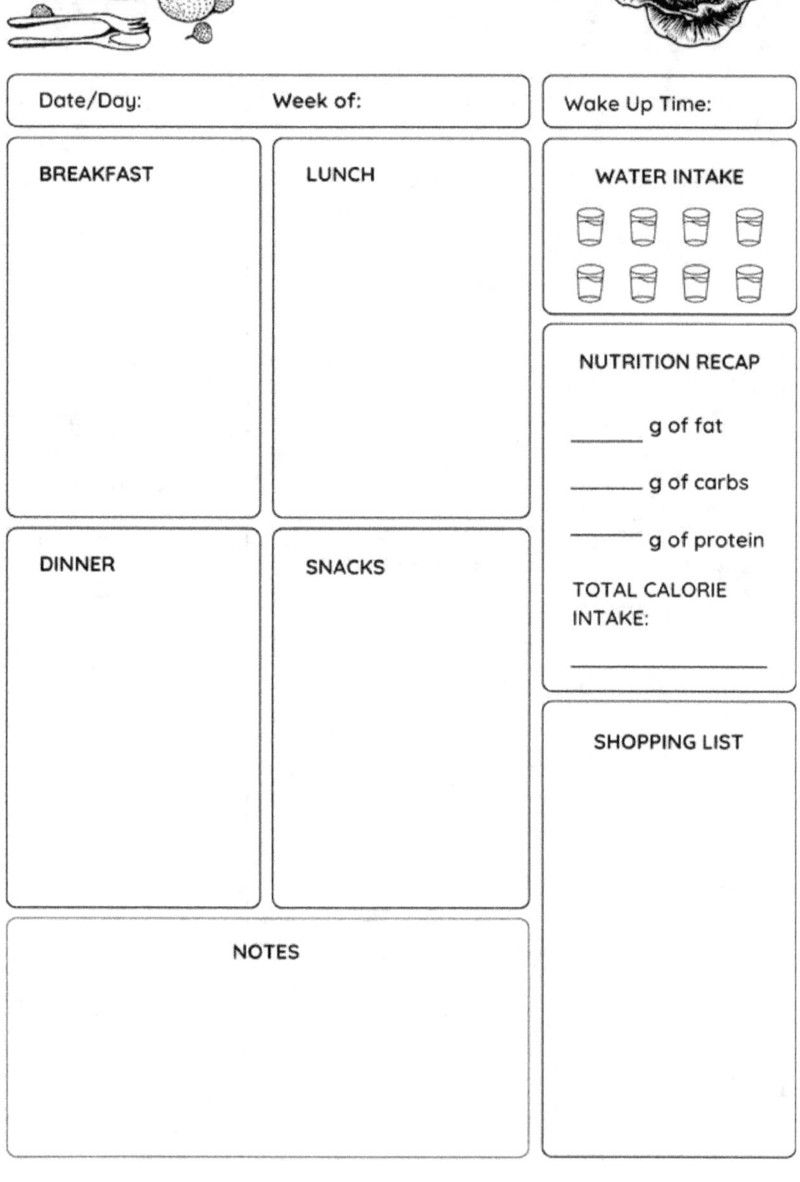

Date/Day: Week of: Wake Up Time:

BREAKFAST

LUNCH

WATER INTAKE

NUTRITION RECAP

_______ g of fat

_______ g of carbs

_______ g of protein

TOTAL CALORIE INTAKE:

____

DINNER

SNACKS

SHOPPING LIST

NOTES

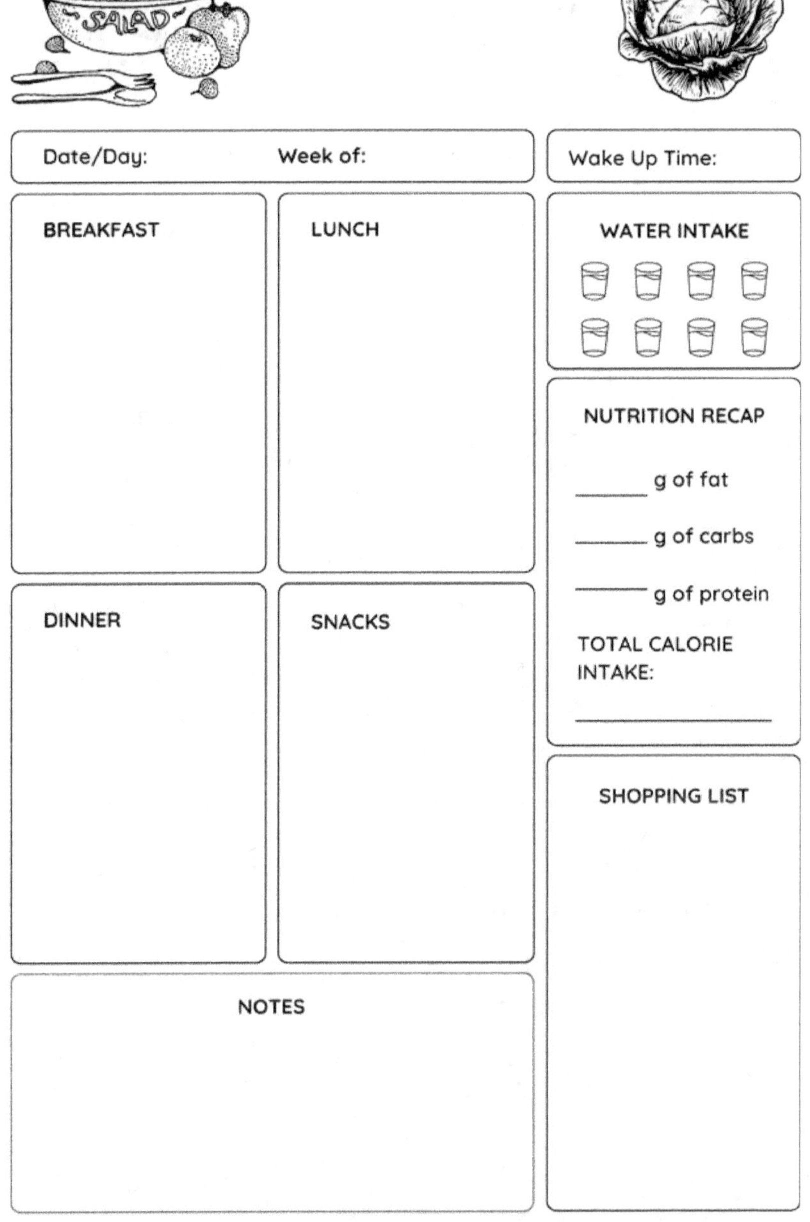

Date/Day: Week of:

Wake Up Time:

BREAKFAST

LUNCH

WATER INTAKE

NUTRITION RECAP

_______ g of fat

_______ g of carbs

_______ g of protein

TOTAL CALORIE INTAKE:

____

DINNER

SNACKS

SHOPPING LIST

NOTES

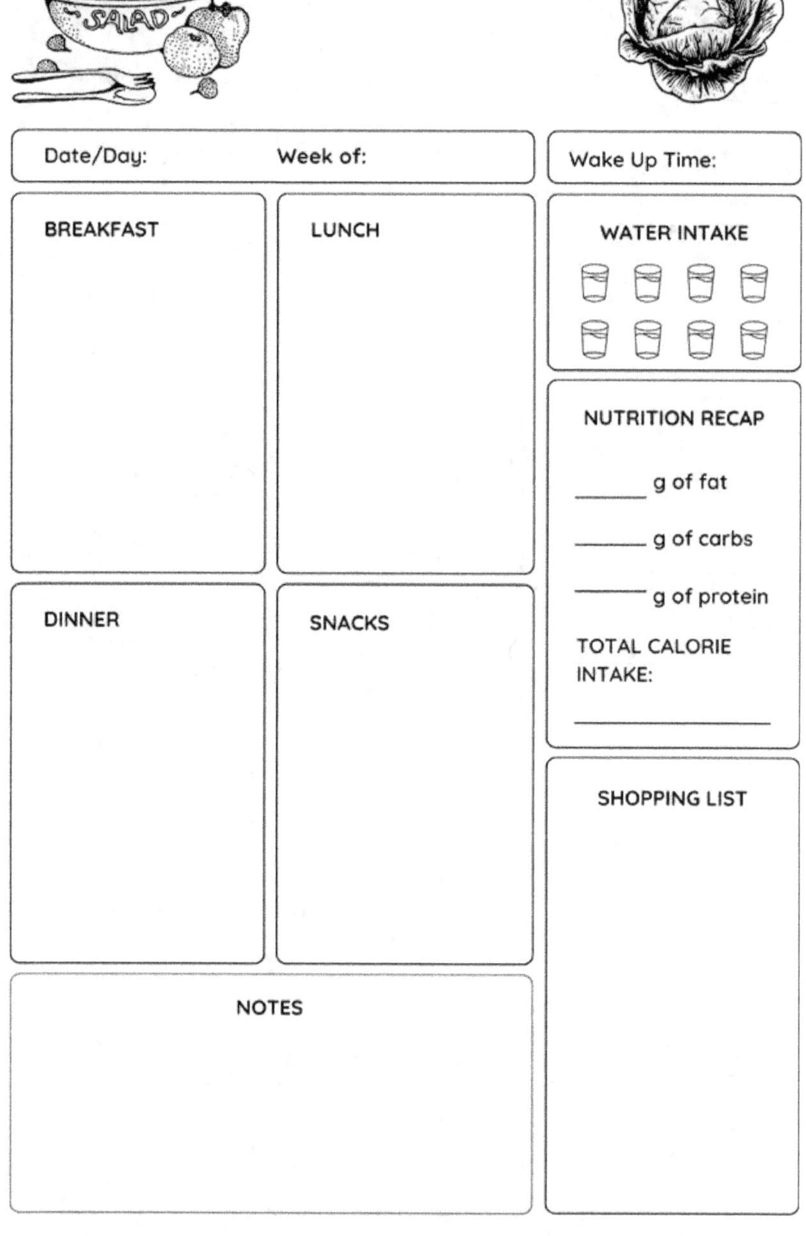

| Date/Day: | Week of: | Wake Up Time: |

BREAKFAST

LUNCH

WATER INTAKE

NUTRITION RECAP

_________ g of fat

_________ g of carbs

_________ g of protein

TOTAL CALORIE INTAKE:

____

DINNER

SNACKS

SHOPPING LIST

NOTES

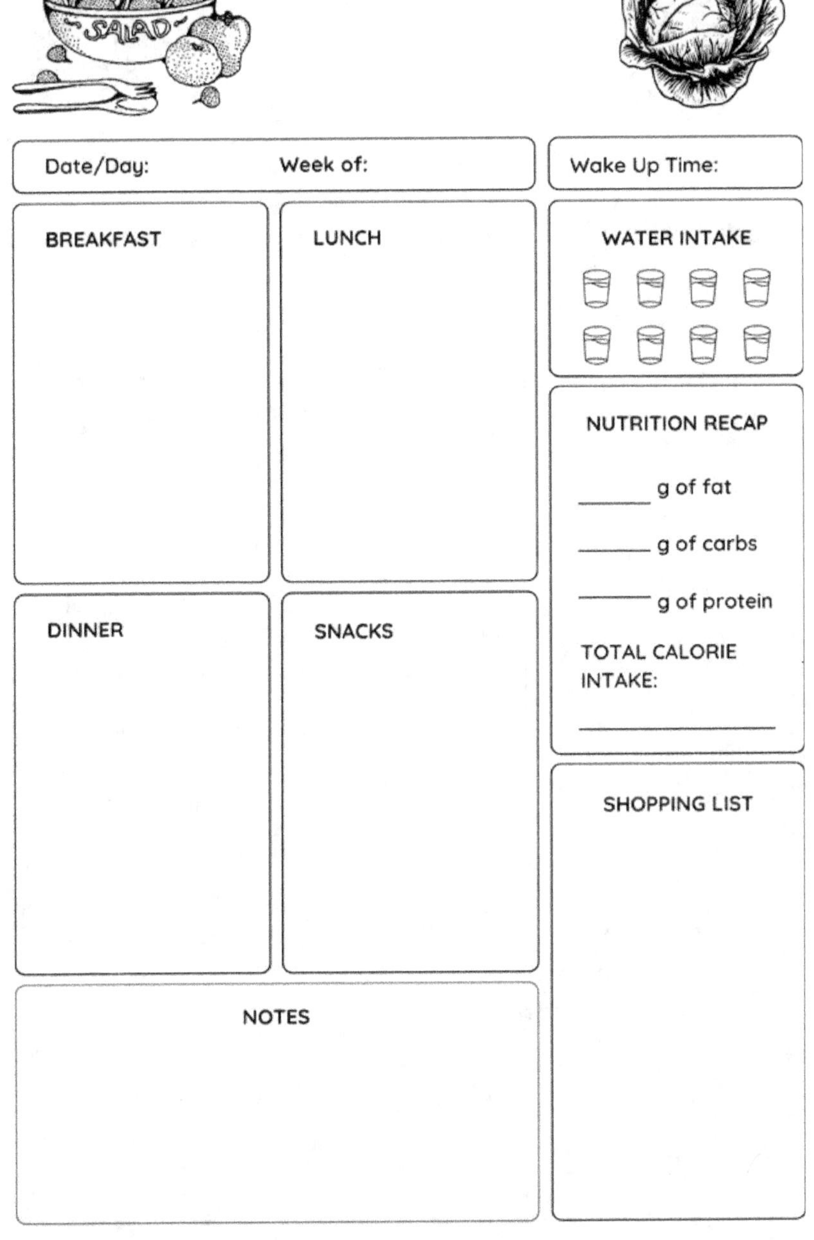

| Date/Day: | Week of: | Wake Up Time: |

BREAKFAST

LUNCH

WATER INTAKE

NUTRITION RECAP

______ g of fat

______ g of carbs

______ g of protein

TOTAL CALORIE INTAKE:

DINNER

SNACKS

SHOPPING LIST

NOTES

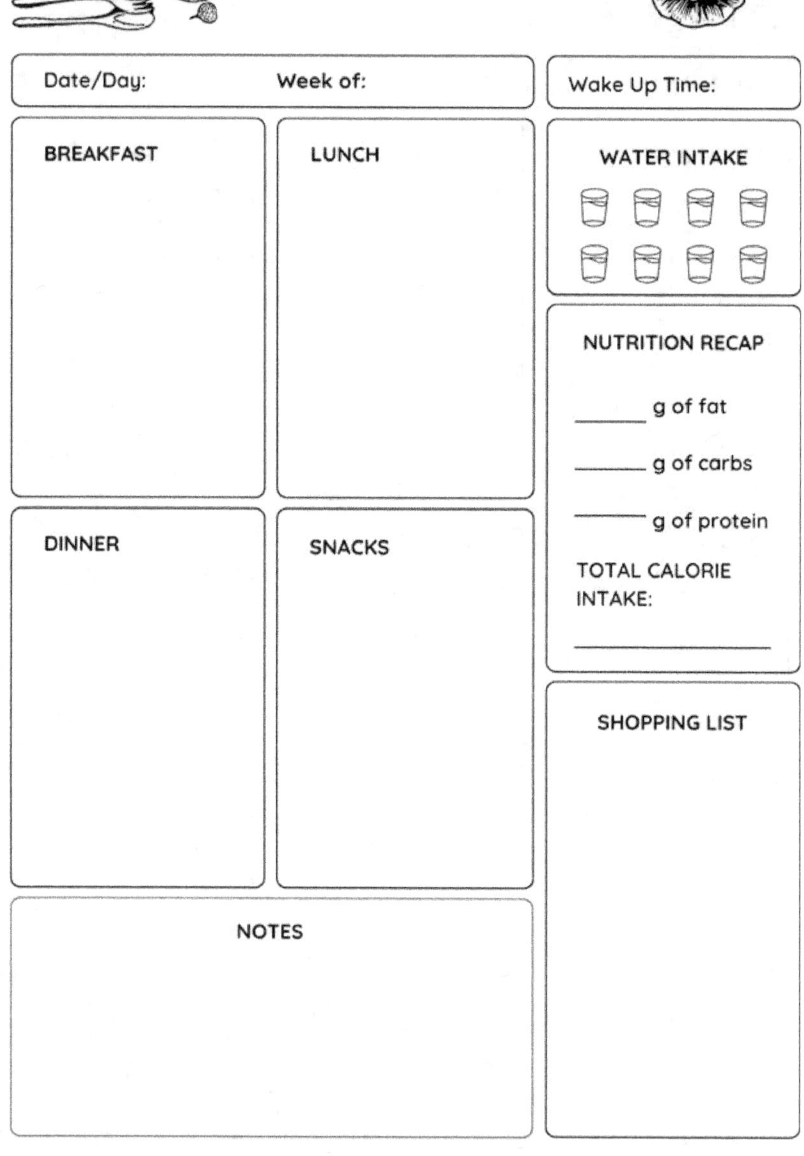

Date/Day: Week of:
Wake Up Time:
BREAKFAST
LUNCH
WATER INTAKE
NUTRITION RECAP
_______ g of fat
_______ g of carbs
_______ g of protein
TOTAL CALORIE INTAKE:
DINNER
SNACKS
SHOPPING LIST
NOTES

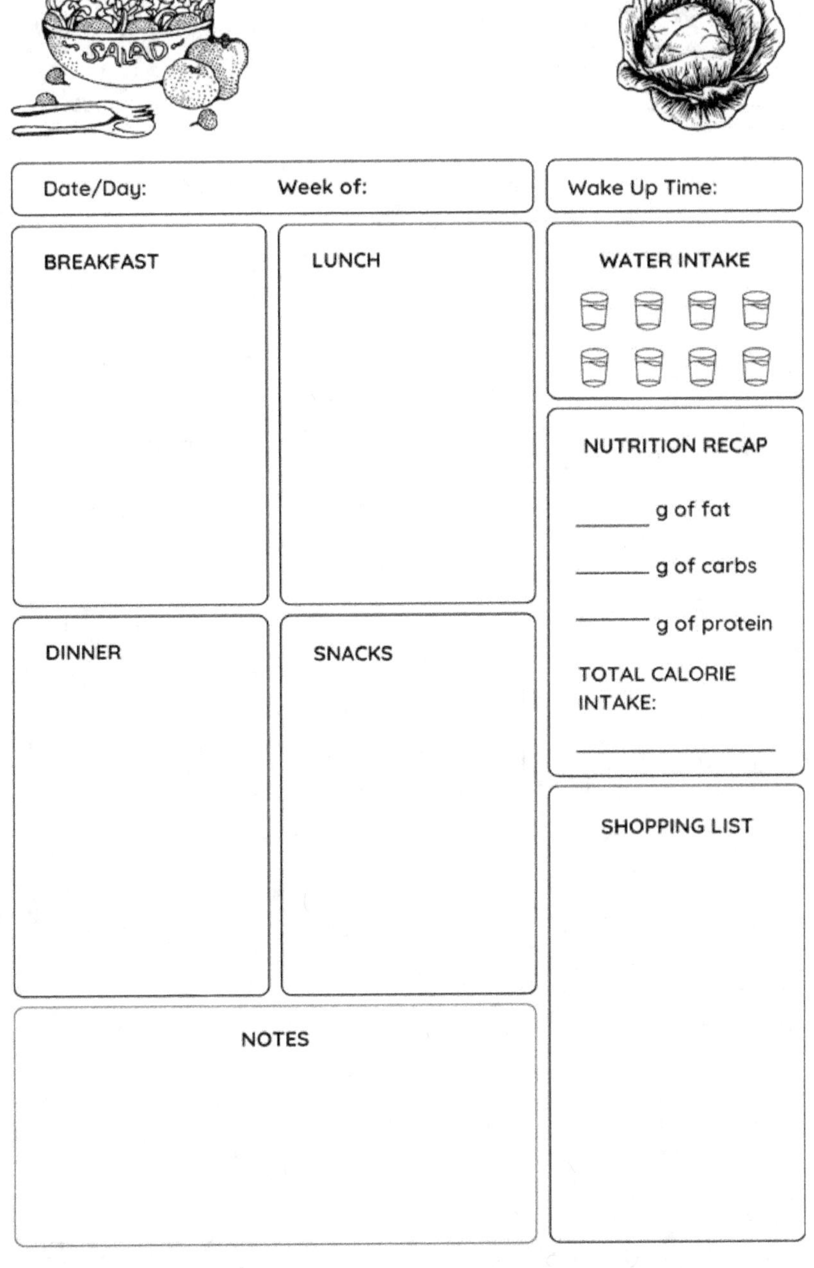

Date/Day:
Week of:
Wake Up Time:
BREAKFAST
LUNCH
WATER INTAKE
NUTRITION RECAP
_______ g of fat
_______ g of carbs
_______ g of protein
TOTAL CALORIE INTAKE:
____
DINNER
SNACKS
SHOPPING LIST
NOTES

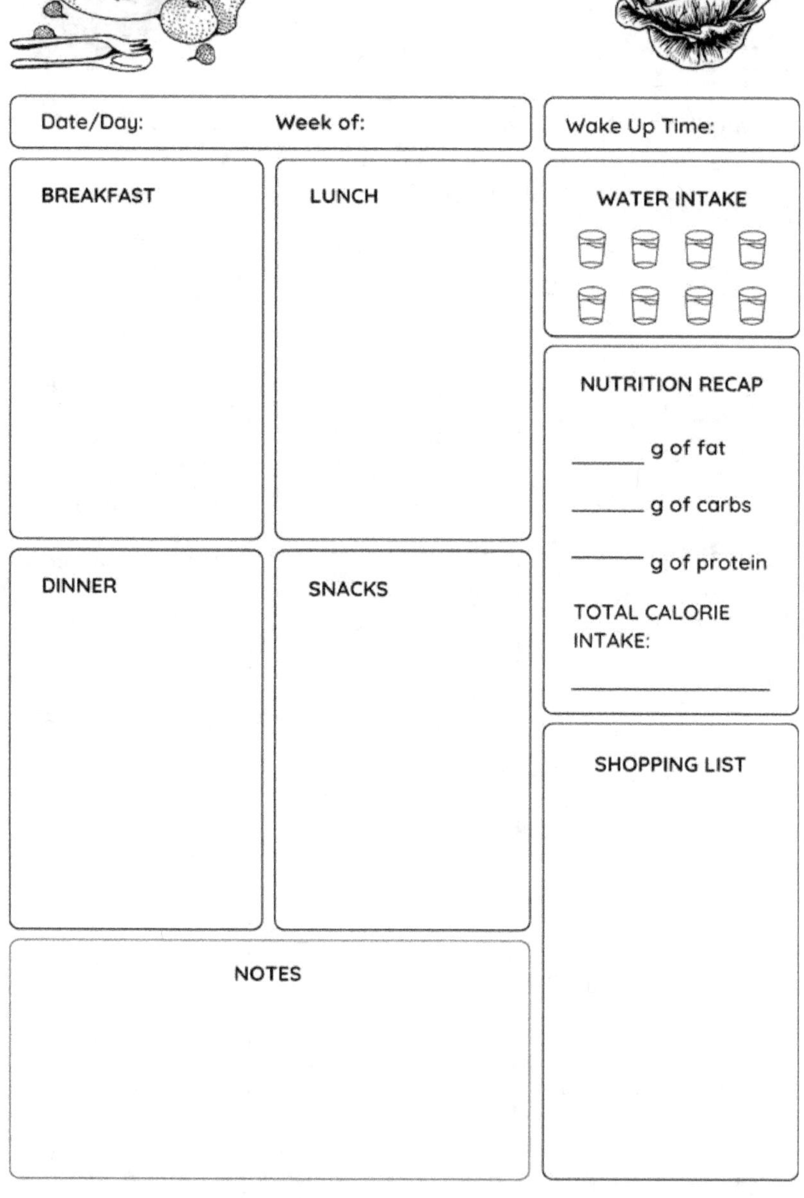

Date/Day: Week of:

Wake Up Time:

BREAKFAST

LUNCH

WATER INTAKE

NUTRITION RECAP

_______ g of fat

_______ g of carbs

_______ g of protein

TOTAL CALORIE INTAKE:

____

DINNER

SNACKS

SHOPPING LIST

NOTES

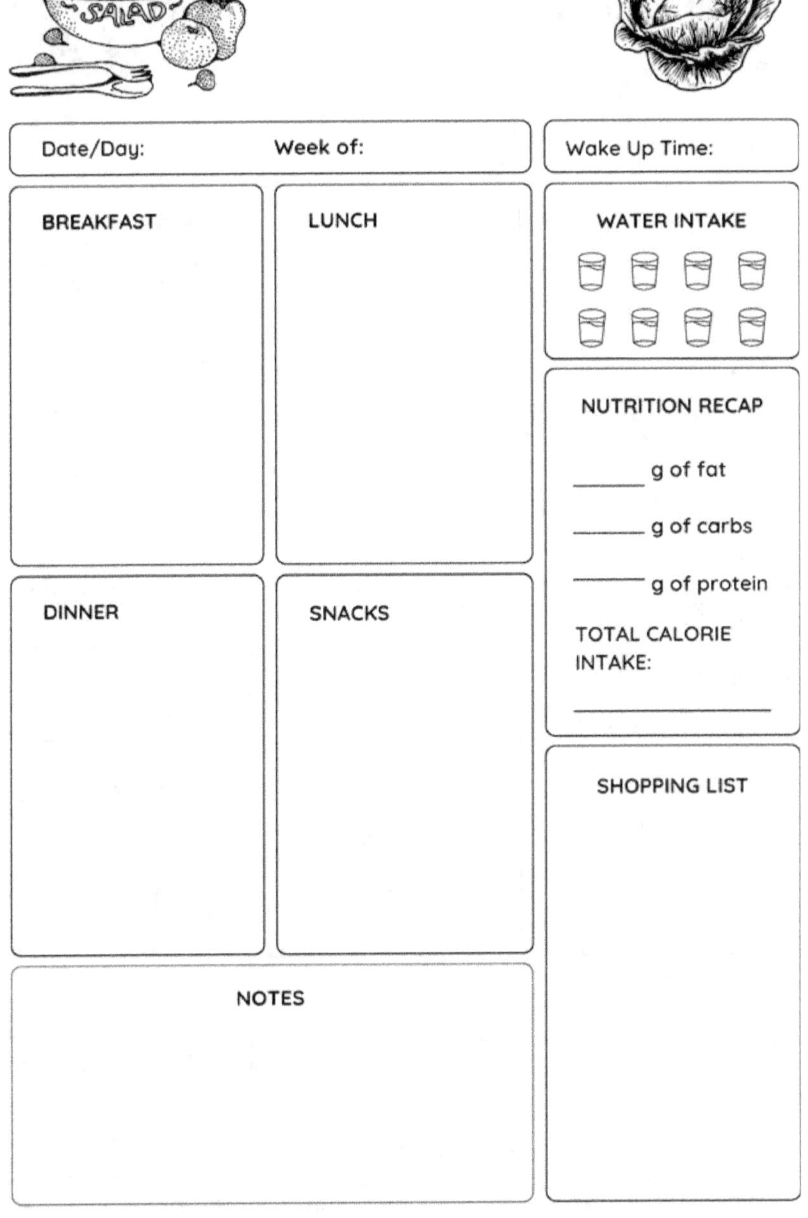

Date/Day: Week of:

Wake Up Time:

BREAKFAST

LUNCH

WATER INTAKE

NUTRITION RECAP

_______ g of fat

_______ g of carbs

_______ g of protein

TOTAL CALORIE INTAKE:

____

DINNER

SNACKS

SHOPPING LIST

NOTES

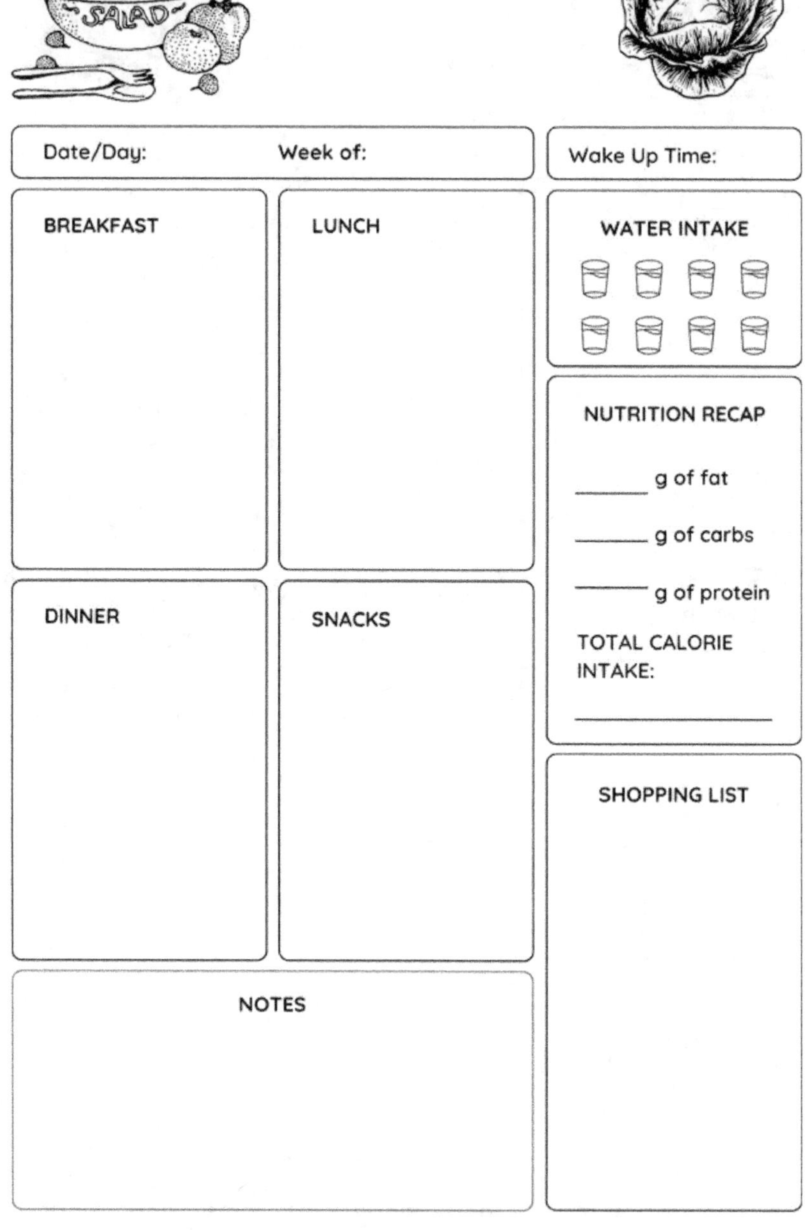

| Date/Day: | Week of: | Wake Up Time: |

BREAKFAST

LUNCH

WATER INTAKE

NUTRITION RECAP

_______ g of fat

_______ g of carbs

_______ g of protein

TOTAL CALORIE INTAKE:

____

DINNER

SNACKS

SHOPPING LIST

NOTES

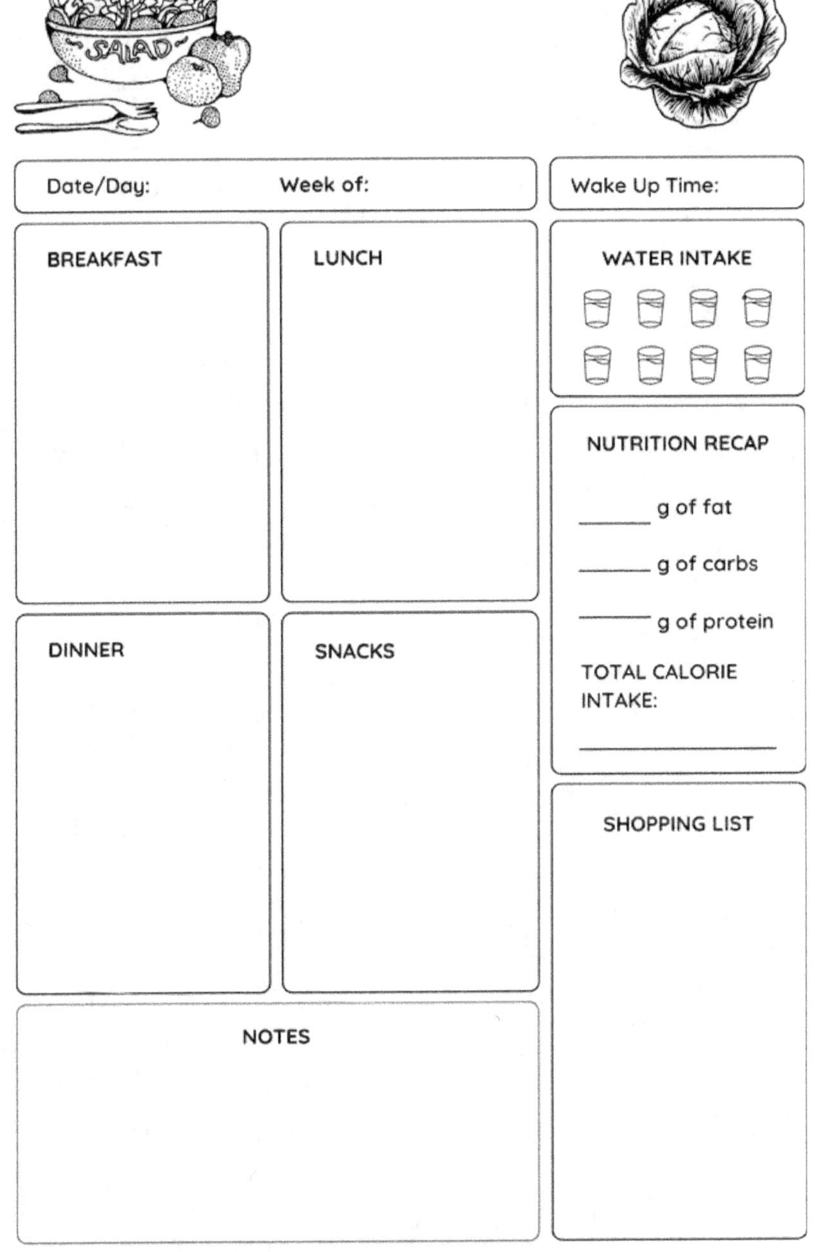

Date/Day:
Week of:
Wake Up Time:
BREAKFAST
LUNCH
WATER INTAKE
NUTRITION RECAP
_______ g of fat
_______ g of carbs
_______ g of protein
TOTAL CALORIE INTAKE:
DINNER
SNACKS
SHOPPING LIST
NOTES

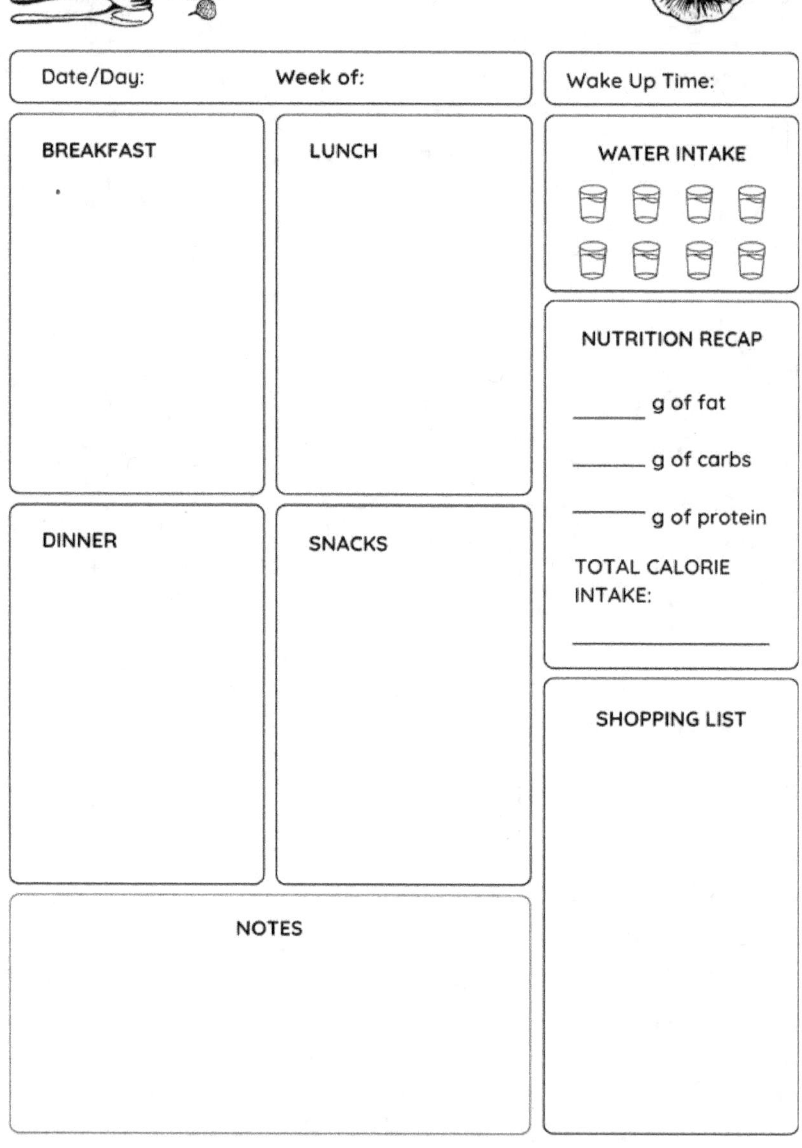

Date/Day: Week of:

Wake Up Time:

BREAKFAST

LUNCH

WATER INTAKE

NUTRITION RECAP

________ g of fat

________ g of carbs

________ g of protein

TOTAL CALORIE INTAKE:

____

DINNER

SNACKS

SHOPPING LIST

NOTES

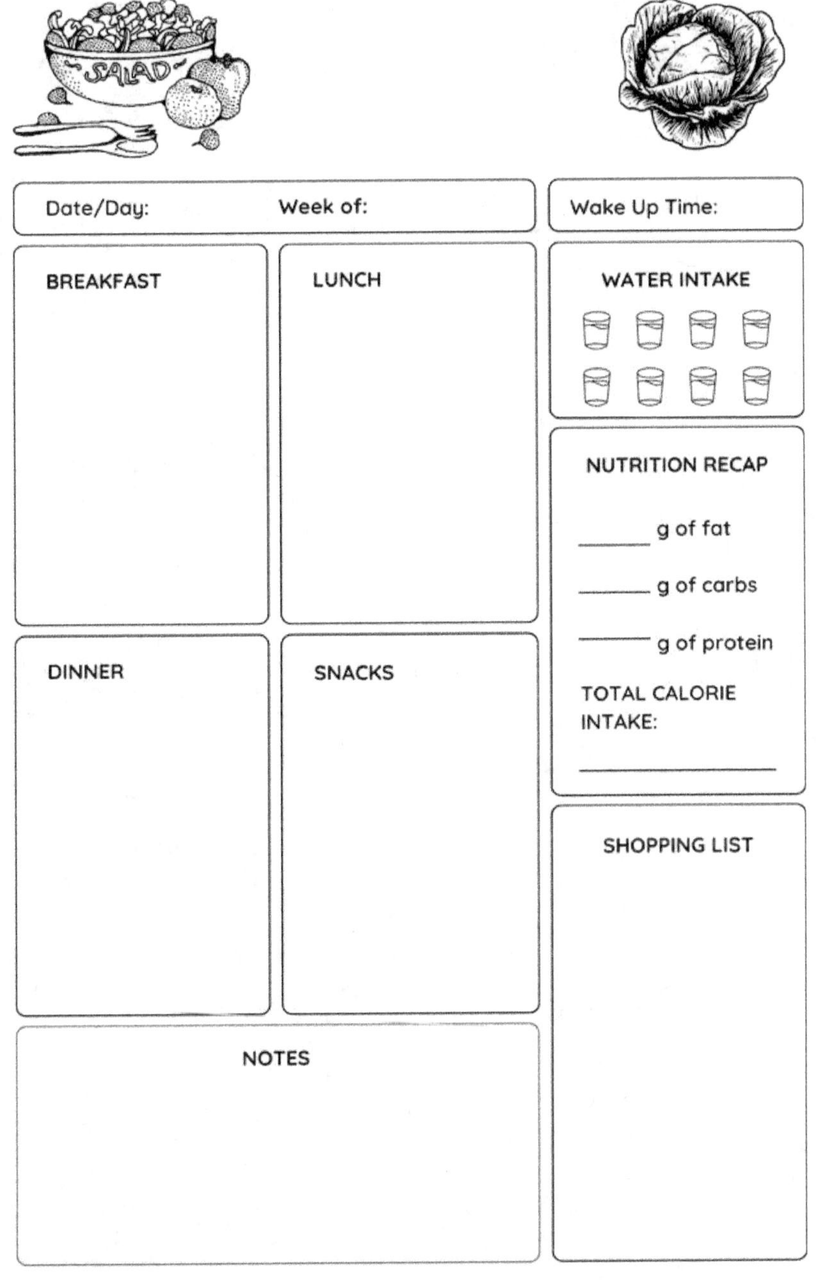

| Date/Day: | Week of: | Wake Up Time: |

BREAKFAST

LUNCH

WATER INTAKE

NUTRITION RECAP

_______ g of fat

_______ g of carbs

_______ g of protein

TOTAL CALORIE INTAKE:

____

DINNER

SNACKS

SHOPPING LIST

NOTES

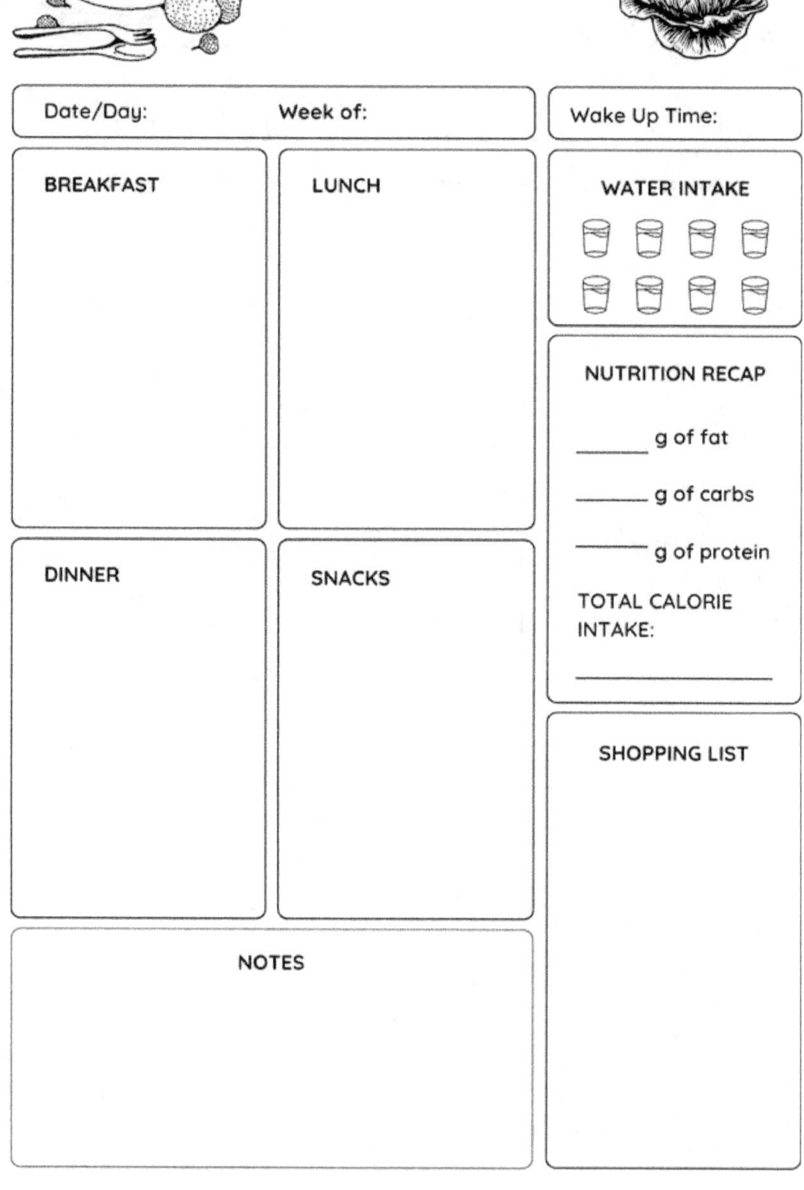

Date/Day: Week of:

Wake Up Time:

BREAKFAST

LUNCH

WATER INTAKE

NUTRITION RECAP

________ g of fat

________ g of carbs

________ g of protein

TOTAL CALORIE INTAKE:

____

DINNER

SNACKS

SHOPPING LIST

NOTES

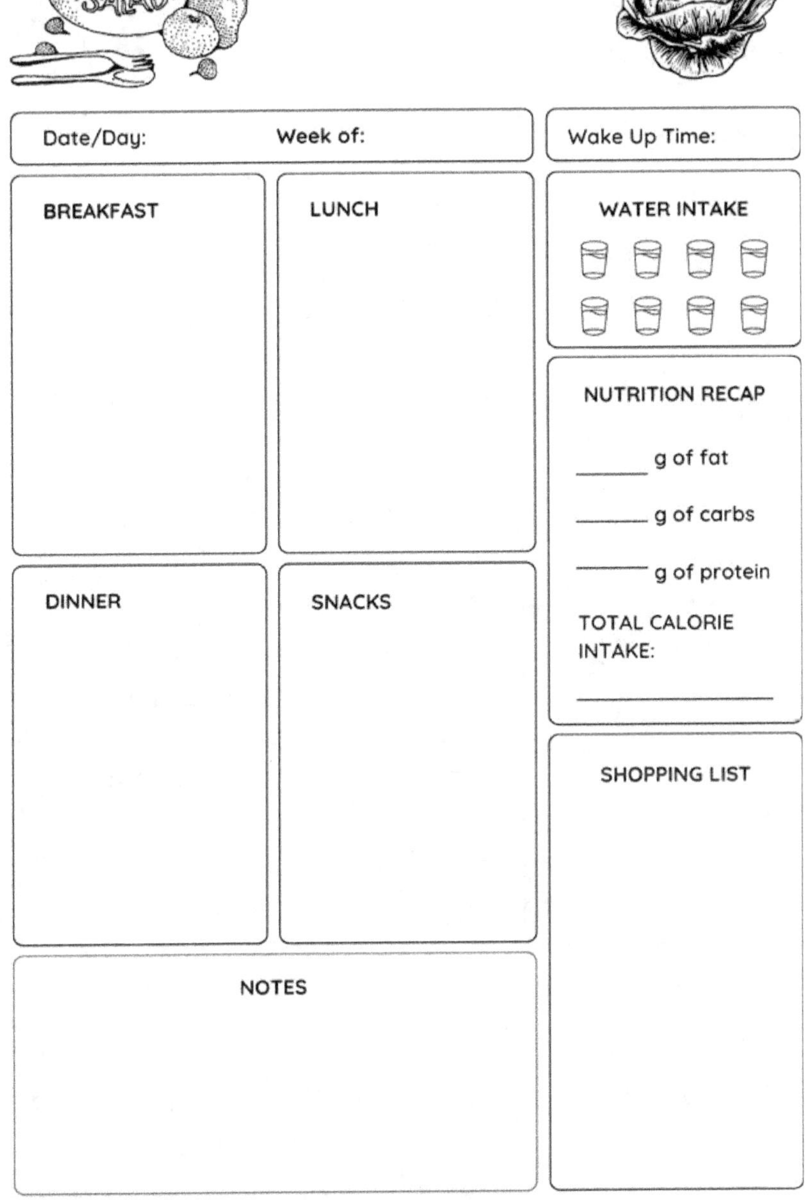

Date/Day:
Week of:
Wake Up Time:
BREAKFAST
LUNCH
WATER INTAKE
NUTRITION RECAP
_______ g of fat
_______ g of carbs
_______ g of protein
TOTAL CALORIE
INTAKE:
DINNER
SNACKS
SHOPPING LIST
NOTES

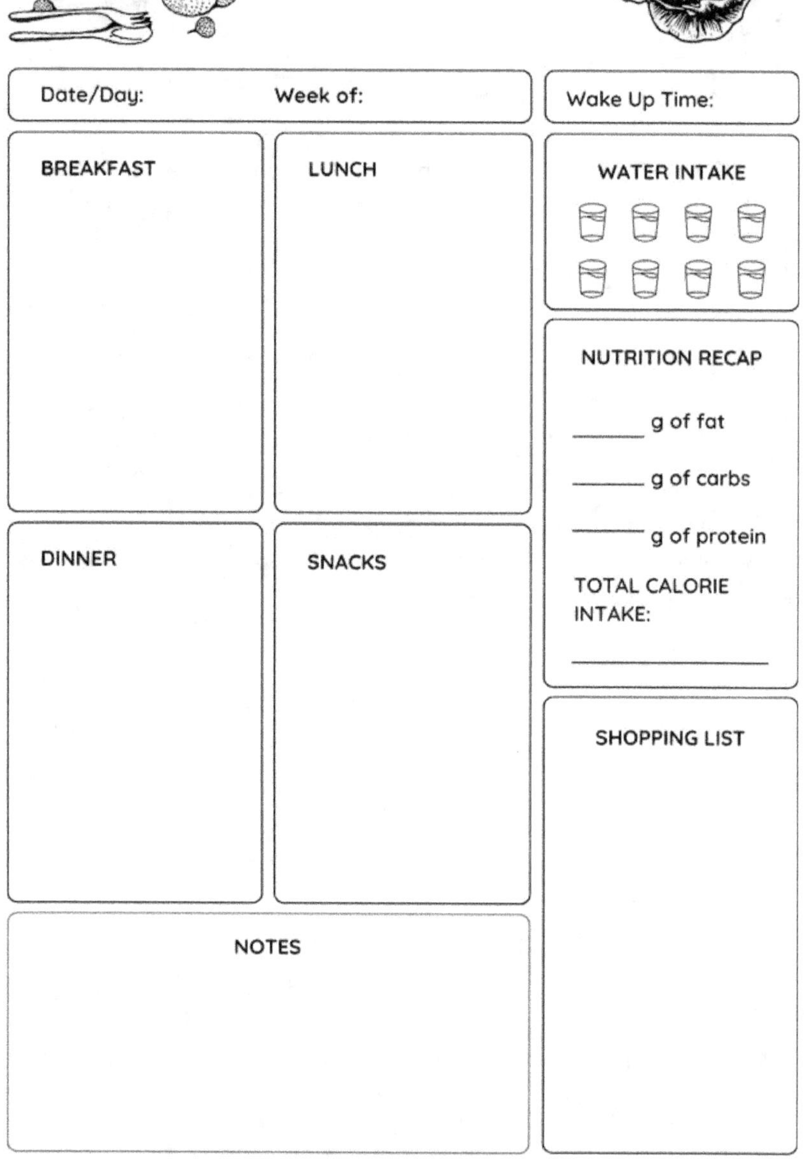

Date/Day: | Week of:

Wake Up Time:

BREAKFAST

LUNCH

WATER INTAKE

DINNER

SNACKS

NUTRITION RECAP

_________ g of fat

_________ g of carbs

_________ g of protein

TOTAL CALORIE INTAKE:

____

SHOPPING LIST

NOTES

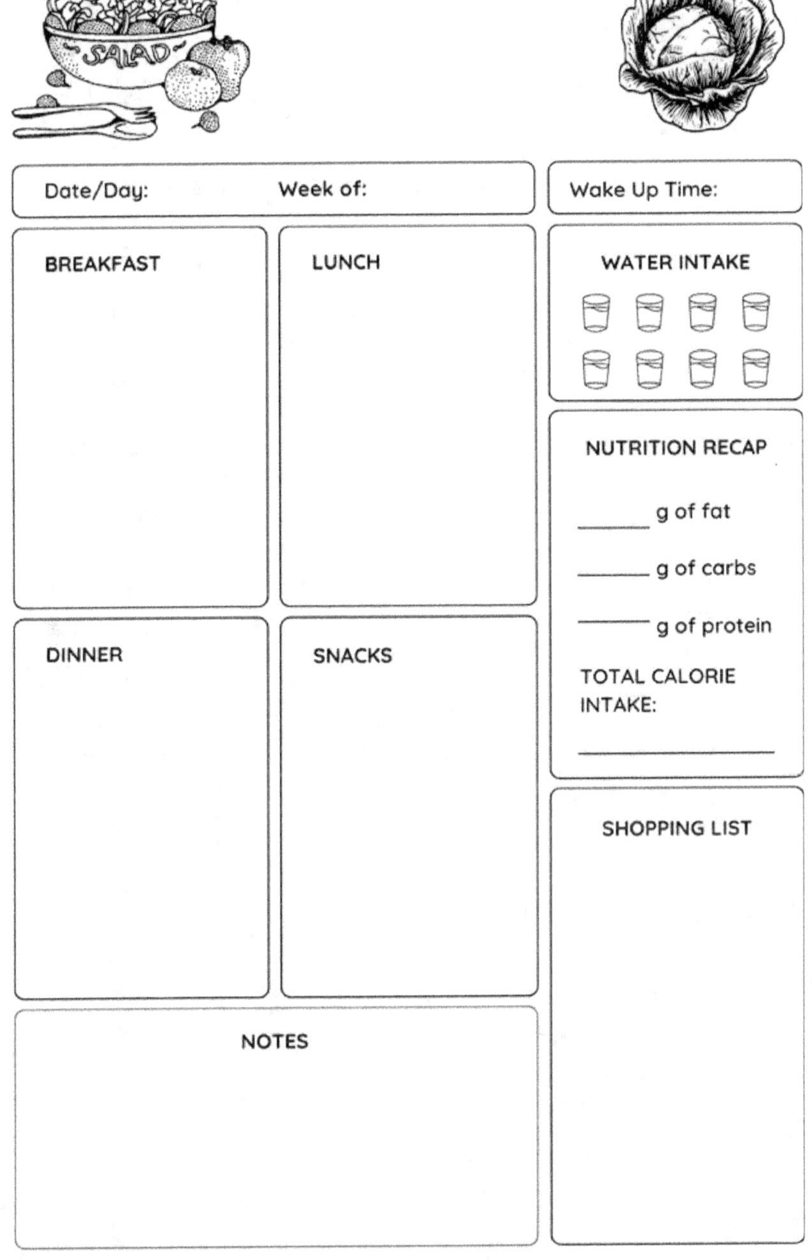

| Date/Day: | Week of: | Wake Up Time: |

BREAKFAST

LUNCH

WATER INTAKE

NUTRITION RECAP

_________ g of fat

_________ g of carbs

_________ g of protein

TOTAL CALORIE INTAKE:

____

DINNER

SNACKS

SHOPPING LIST

NOTES

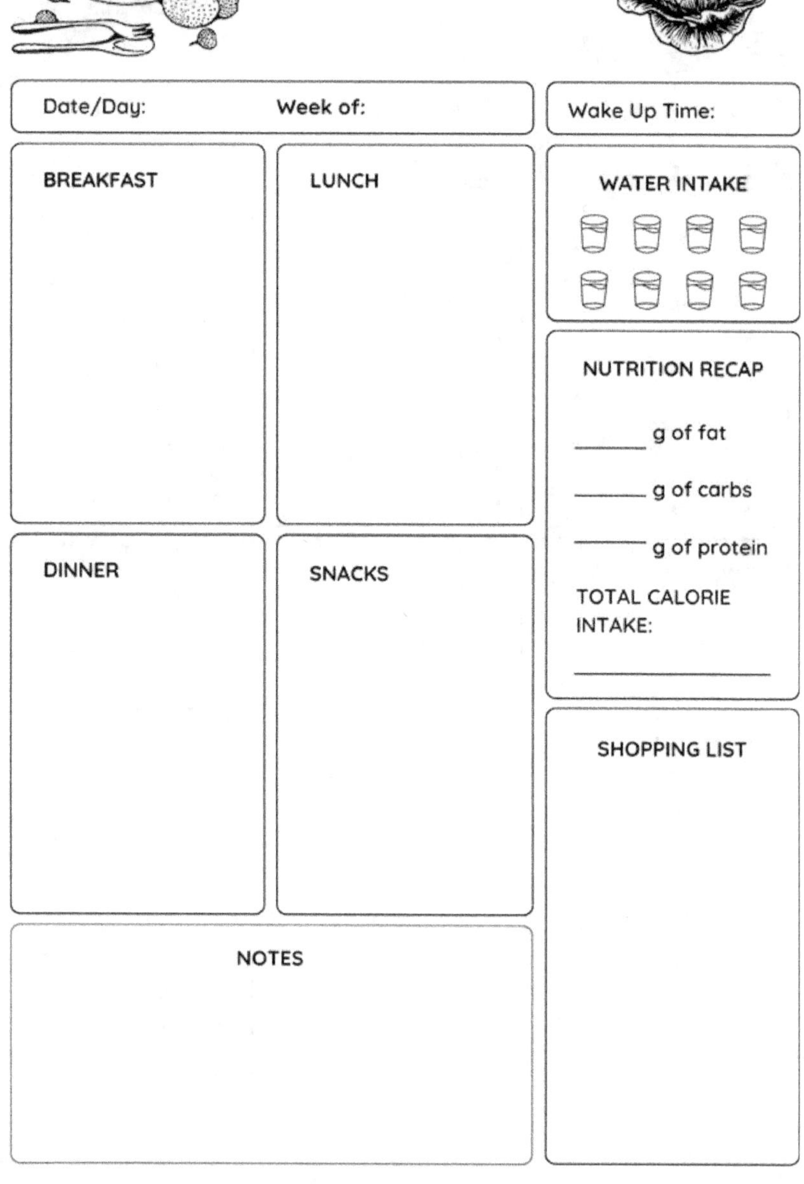

| Date/Day: | Week of: | Wake Up Time: |

BREAKFAST

LUNCH

WATER INTAKE

NUTRITION RECAP

_______ g of fat

_______ g of carbs

_______ g of protein

TOTAL CALORIE INTAKE:

____

DINNER

SNACKS

SHOPPING LIST

NOTES

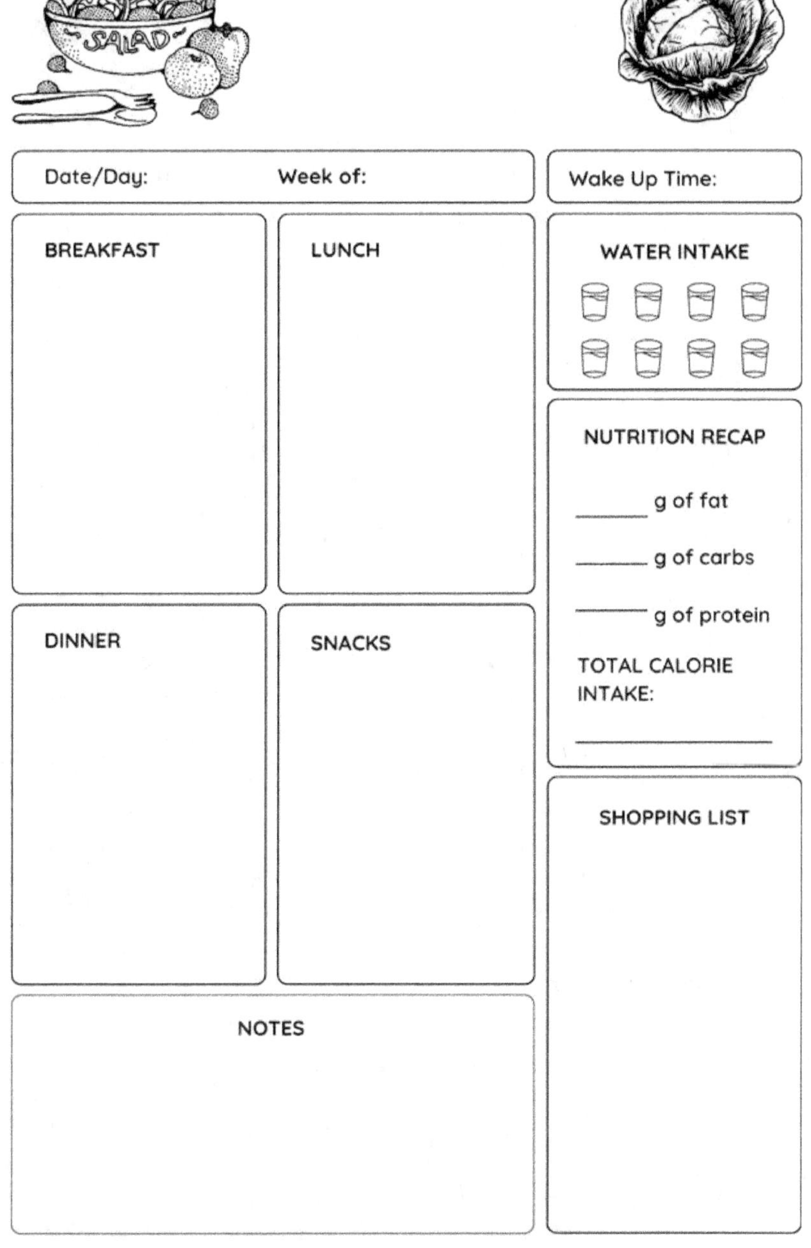

Date/Day: Week of:

Wake Up Time:

BREAKFAST

LUNCH

WATER INTAKE

NUTRITION RECAP

_______ g of fat

_______ g of carbs

_______ g of protein

TOTAL CALORIE INTAKE:

____

DINNER

SNACKS

SHOPPING LIST

NOTES

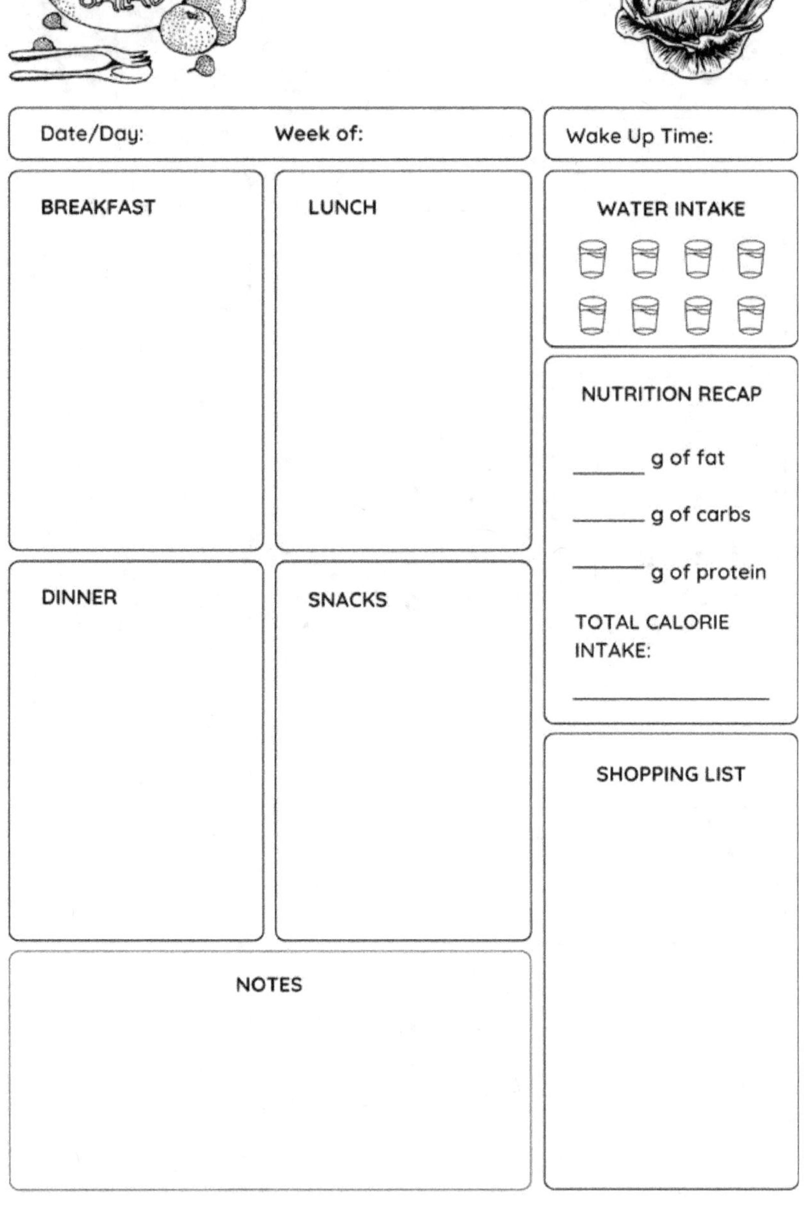

Date/Day:
Week of:
Wake Up Time:
BREAKFAST
LUNCH
WATER INTAKE
NUTRITION RECAP
_______ g of fat
_______ g of carbs
_______ g of protein
TOTAL CALORIE INTAKE:
DINNER
SNACKS
SHOPPING LIST
NOTES

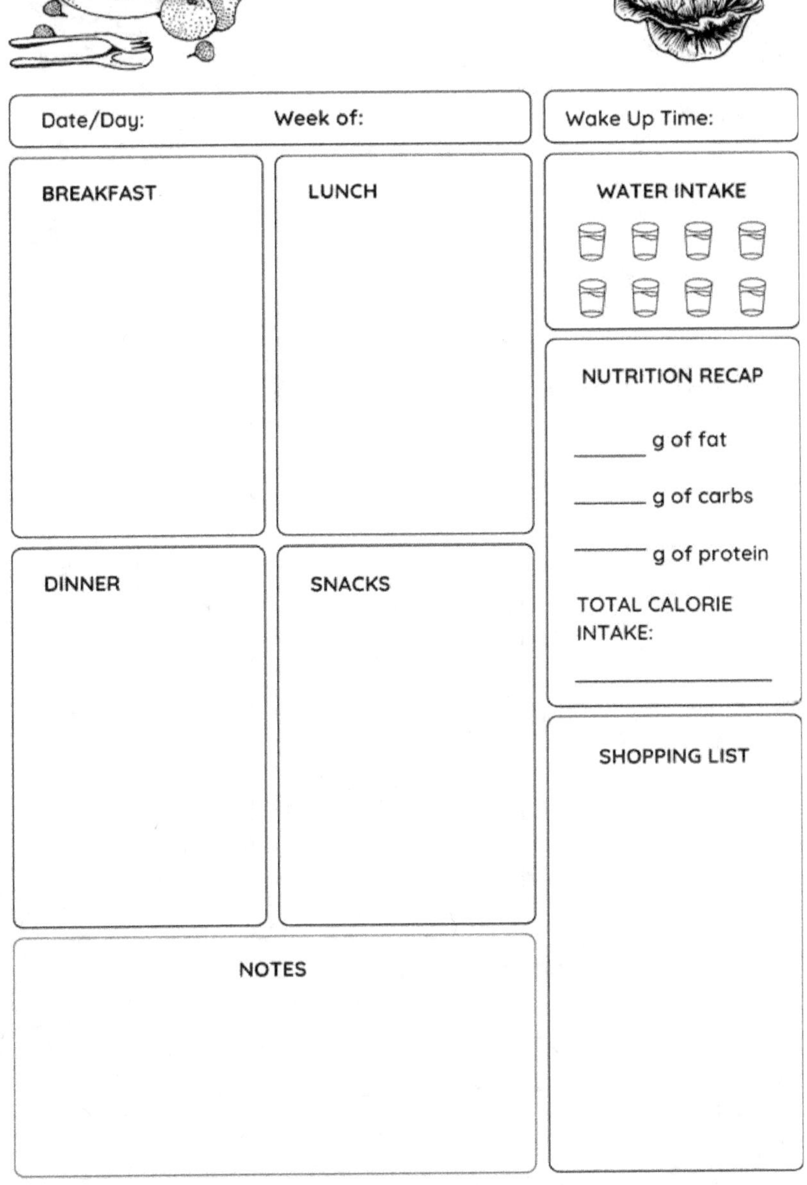

Date/Day:
Week of:
Wake Up Time:
BREAKFAST
LUNCH
WATER INTAKE
NUTRITION RECAP
_______ g of fat
_______ g of carbs
_______ g of protein
TOTAL CALORIE INTAKE:
DINNER
SNACKS
SHOPPING LIST
NOTES

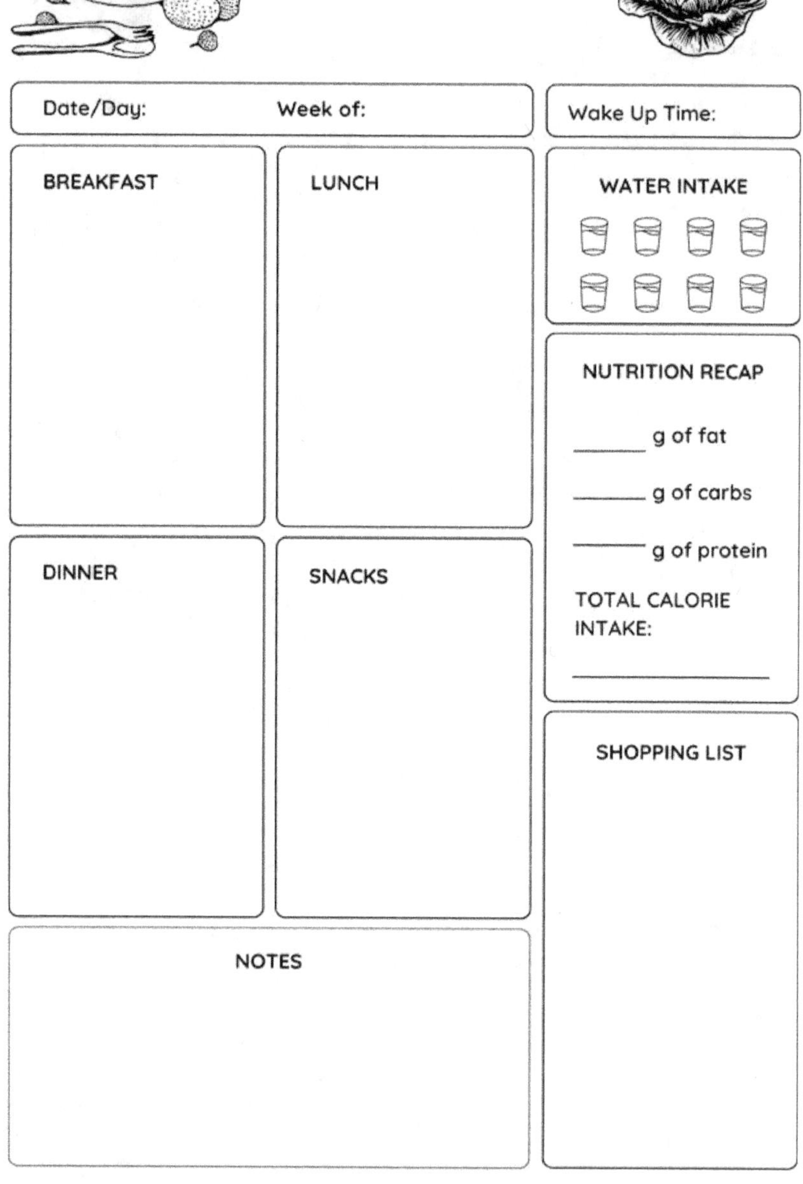

Date/Day: Week of:

Wake Up Time:

BREAKFAST

LUNCH

WATER INTAKE

NUTRITION RECAP

________ g of fat

________ g of carbs

________ g of protein

TOTAL CALORIE INTAKE:

____

DINNER

SNACKS

SHOPPING LIST

NOTES

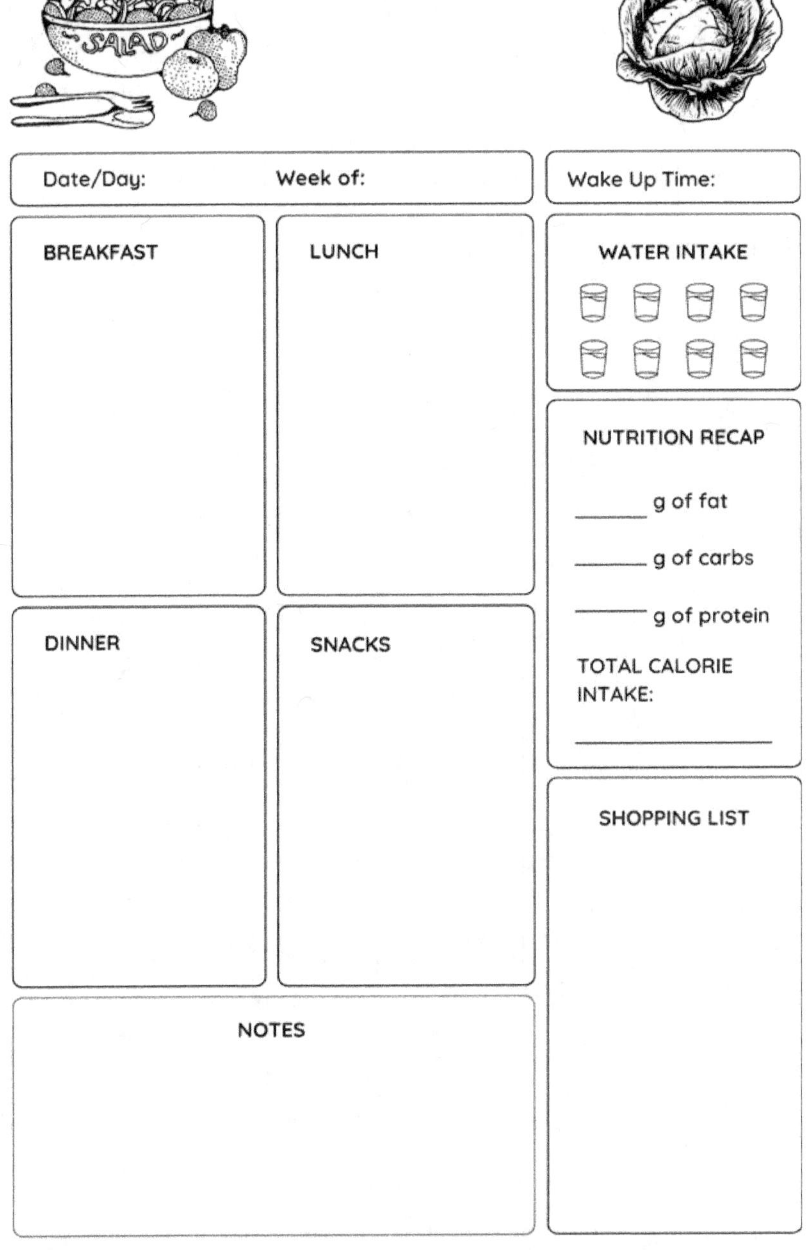

Date/Day: Week of:

Wake Up Time:

BREAKFAST

LUNCH

WATER INTAKE

NUTRITION RECAP

_________ g of fat

_________ g of carbs

_________ g of protein

TOTAL CALORIE INTAKE:

____

DINNER

SNACKS

SHOPPING LIST

NOTES

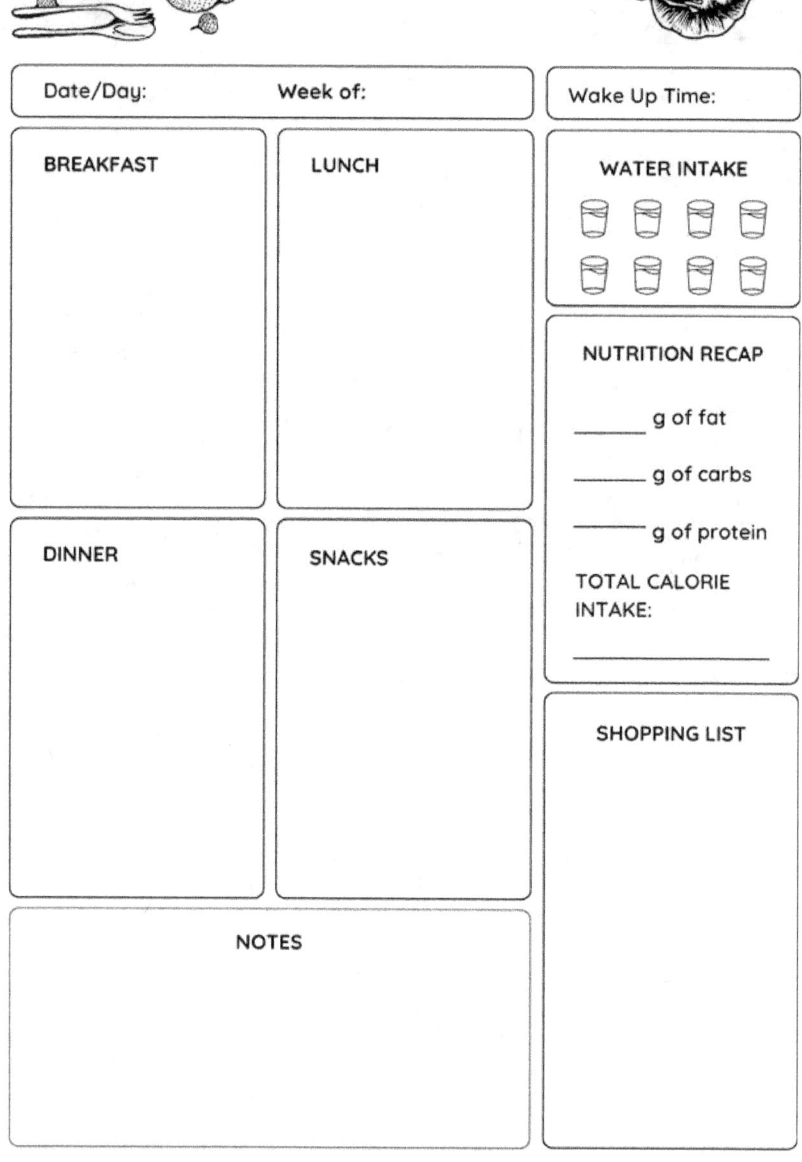

Date/Day: Week of:

Wake Up Time:

BREAKFAST

LUNCH

WATER INTAKE

NUTRITION RECAP

_______ g of fat

_______ g of carbs

_______ g of protein

TOTAL CALORIE
INTAKE:

____

DINNER

SNACKS

SHOPPING LIST

NOTES